Why Am I So Exhausted?

understanding chronic fatigue syndrome

To dear Maggie, my long-suffering wife, without whose patience, support and computer skills this book would not have been written. Apologies to Sophie our rescue Spanish Greyhound/Galgo for all those long boring days whilst we worked; at least she was in front of the fire.

Why Am I So Exhausted?

understanding chronic fatigue syndrome

Martin Budd

Hammersmith Health Books

London

First published in 2013 by Hammersmith Health Books – an imprint of Hammersmith Books Limited
14 Greville Street, London EC1N 8SB, UK
www.hammersmithbooks.co.uk

Disclaimer

Whilst the advice and information in this book are believed to be true and accurate at the date of going to press, neither the author nor the publisher can accept any legal responsibility or liability for any errors or omissions that may be made.

Tests: The various tests described in this book can only be requested by a practitioner. The laboratories insist on a completed test request from a practitioner with the blood, urine or saliva samples.

Supplements: Many of the supplements, in particular the glandulars, described in this book also require a practitioner's prescription and order form. They are *not* for over-the-counter sales.

British Library Cataloguing in Publication Data: A CIP record of this book is available from the British Library.

Print ISBN: 978-1-78161-023-7
Ebook ISBN: 978-1-78161-024-4

Commissioning editor: Georgina Bentliff
Designed and typeset by: Phoenix Photosetting, Chatham, Kent
Index: Dr Laurence Errington
Production: Helen Whitehorn, Pathmedia
Printed and bound by TJ International
Cover image: Shutterstock Images

Contents

Contents

Preface

•

Even before my first book (*Low Blood Sugar*) in 1981, I had a special interest in diagnosing and treating fatigue. As I will describe in this, my latest book, fatigue is the symptom we experience most frequently, after pain.

It was during the early '80s that I became aware of the huge diversity of causes of human fatigue. I was very fortunate to be invited to join a specialised clinic in Basingstoke and become one of the directors. With five practitioners, including a medical doctor, a medical herbalist, two naturopaths and an acupuncturist, we were able to employ a full-time biochemist to do our blood testing. The director of the clinic was Keith Lamont, who also founded and acted as Dean of the College of Acupuncture for several years.

It was during my involvement with the Basingstoke Clinic that I developed an interest in the causes of chronic fatigue, including hypothyroidism, low blood sugar, iron-deficient anaemia and many peripheral conditions that I describe in this book.

Over the intervening years I have written three books on low blood sugar and a book on diabetic diets; also, *Diets to help Migraine* and *Why Can't I Lose Weight?* My wife Maggie has assisted me with the recipes in these books. However, in 2000, my interest in fatigue became more focused and I wrote *Why Am I So Tired?* which describes a non-medical treatment approach to hypothyroidism.

Not surprisingly, the sale of these books brought many very tired patients to my door and I was able to develop a specialised practice diagnosing and treating the many causes of fatigue. I continue to see patients in Hampshire and central London.

This latest book draws on those years of general and specialist experience and will, I hope, encourage you, the reader, to realise that chronic fatigue is frequently the result of several causes. If you and your practitioner(s) have been looking for a single cause and treatment, you will almost certainly have been disappointed. When several contributory causes are involved (and in some of my patients it may be four or five), only a systematic approach to diagnosis and treatment can be effective.

I only hope that the contents of my book will offer optimism and hope to CFS sufferers.

Martin Budd
2013

About the Author

Martin Budd graduated as a Registered Naturopath in 1963 after four years' study and he has practised as a Naturopathic Consultant for 50 years. He practised for some years in Essex and Cheshire, and in the early 1970s he became a Director of the Basingstoke Clinic. This was a multi-therapy facility set up with a laboratory and X-ray unit to offer diagnostic services to patients and practitioners.

It was during this time that Martin developed a special interest in blood sugar disorders and fatigue. This culminated in his first book, *Low Blood Sugar* published in 1981. This was followed by books on diabetes, migraine, hypothyroidism, fatigue and obesity. He also co-authored several recipe books with his wife, Maggie. These books have been variously printed in Spanish, Russian, Italian, Greek, French, Portuguese, Danish, Hungarian and Hebrew. Australian, South African and American editions have also been published.

With the publication of these books and his lecturing, Martin has become an authority on the diagnosis and treatment of blood sugar disorders, hypothyroidism, chronic fatigue syndrome, obesity, stress and allied health problems. Patients travel from many parts of the United Kingdom, Europe and America to his practices in Lymington, Hampshire and London (Harley Street).

Contact details

All correspondence to   Blenheim
                                Priestlands Lane
                                Lymington
                                SO41 8HZ, UK

Telephone contact for both practices: +44 (0)792 687 55 66
Email contact: martinbudd.secretary@yahoo.co.uk

Chapter 1

The history of chronic fatigue syndrome

I must start this book by making it clear what I mean by the terms I use. Throughout I will use the term 'chronic fatigue syndrome' (CFS) to describe severe, long-term exhaustion, *irrespective* of the cause or causes. In this first chapter I will explain why this is and review other labels that have been/ are used to describe conditions that come under the CFS 'umbrella'. My aim is to shed light on what is known about this controversial condition, and what is generally agreed and what is contested. This is important background to the chapters that follow, looking at causes, diagnosis and treatment. To be clear from the start, my 40-plus years of experience as a naturopath specialising in fatigue have taught me that chronic fatigue always has multiple, generally interrelated, causes, all of which need to be treated before health is restored. Indeed, I regularly see patients with four or five overlapping contributory problems.

What is chronic fatigue syndrome?

It can be very reassuring for exhausted patients if their doctor can offer them a diagnosis, thus providing a reason for their symptoms. In medicine, a diagnosis is usually required before treatment commences. Although prescriptions are given to assist symptom-relief, effective treatment for any health problems can only really work with an accurate diagnosis. Herein lies the problem with what is called the 'chronic fatigue syndrome' (CFS) – the variable cluster of symptoms (see chapter 2) dominated by long-term chronic fatigue for which there is currently no agreed cause or simple diagnostic test. Many doctors refuse to believe that their chronically fatigued patients are physically ill, a judgement endorsed by the frequent absence of 'abnormal' test results. Without an acceptable diagnosis for their distressing symptoms, treatment is not offered. Instead patients are prescribed analgesics (pain killers), sleeping tablets, anti-depressants and other drugs to provide a degree of symptom-relief. This has created an unfortunate situation whereby many patients suffer the symptoms of CFS for several years, and without a recognisable medical 'pigeon-hole' they are usually classified as neurotic or even hysterical.

Many attempts have been made over several decades to identify the cause or causes of CFS. A great deal of controversy has surrounded any attempt to agree on a standardised medical definition. There are those who see the problem as a 20th-century condition and claim that it has developed as a result of a combination of new viruses, excessive vaccinations, drug side-effects, environmental pollutants, food additives and other factors that have perverted or damaged the human chemistry. By contrast, many researchers and medical doctors hold the view that chronically fatigued patients have a psychological component to their symptoms and the fatigue should therefore be defined as psychogenic (caused by mental factors) or psychosomatic (strongly influenced by emotional factors). Myalgic encephalomyelitis (ME) (see page 6) and the Gulf War syndrome are two controversial conditions, or groupings of symptoms, that are cited as explanations for CFS. The term 'psychosomatic rheumatism' has been suggested for chronic fatigue with pain. Any evidence linking ME and CFS to a possible biological cause (a virus had been held to blame) was recently shown to be invalid by scientists at Columbia University, whose work indicated previous evidence in favour of a viral cause had rested on faulty test procedures.

To be able precisely to define such a condition must be the Holy Grail for exhausted patients, who understandably want to know what exactly is wrong with them, and therefore what would be an effective and appropriate treatment. Unfortunately, fatigue is a symptom but it is very rarely what health practitioners call a 'sign'. I will explain what is meant by this and why it matters.

Chapter 1

My medical dictionary defines a sign as, 'An indication of the objective evidence of a disease perceived by an examining physician.' (This could, for example, be the characteristic rash seen in chicken pox.) It likewise defines a symptom as, 'Any *subjective* evidence of a patient's condition, such evidence or sensation being perceived *by the patient*' [my italics].

When a doctor is consulted, the patients' signs and symptoms provide vital clues to a possible diagnosis. CFS is a diagnostic challenge largely because the symptoms are so variable – I have yet to see two patients with identical symptoms – yet signs are rare or non-existent.

Medical testing (blood tests, scans and X-rays etc) can often accurately confirm and identify the severity rating for a patient's symptoms. Such information serves to point to a possible diagnosis for, say, cancer symptoms, digestive disorders, heart and lung conditions and endocrine (hormonal) imbalances. Fatigue, however, is not always easy to measure, and it can therefore be very difficult to assess its severity. Such symptoms as anxiety, irritability and depression are equally difficult to evaluate.

Many exhausted patients look exhausted – that is, they look pale and drawn, their posture is slumped and they can even be tearful, confused and forgetful when discussing their symptoms. These are observable and very useful signs, but I need to know how they themselves define fatigue. Information on the duration and severity of their symptoms is essential in aiding a possible diagnosis and any future treatment strategies.

One of the first questions that I ask my CFS patients at their initial consultation is, 'How do you know that you are fatigued?' This question is often not well received. I assume that they think it a strange request from a practitioner who treats CFS on a regular basis. Responses to my question can be surprising and tend to fall into two groups:

Group 1: These patients can clearly and accurately remember the onset of their symptoms. Some patients can recall almost to the day when their chronic fatigue started. Usually, the symptoms were triggered by a well-remembered event, such as a severe infection, loss of employment, childbirth, major surgery, death of a family member or another unusual stress. This can even include getting married – stress can result from happy events. The important element in this type of response is that the duration of symptoms can be established, because the patient can remember their good health before the onset of the fatigue. This comparison also provides a useful severity rating.

Group 2: These patients simply cannot remember what it is like to be fatigue-free, vital and relaxed. They wake up each day with muscle/joint pain and stiffness and are unrefreshed after eight to 10 hours of sleep. Such symptoms are routine and familiar.

I frequently see people with CFS who have suffered symptoms since puberty, and they consult me aged 30–40 years; likewise, women who have 'never felt well' since their first pregnancy 15–20 years earlier. Other common triggers include glandular fever as a teenager, or food poisoning in Asia during a 'gap year' many years previously. Such patients tend to reply to my question, 'How do you know that you are fatigued?' with an answer based on comparison with family members, friends and work colleagues. Alarm bells ring when you need to go to bed at 9 pm while your friends can't wait to go out for a meal or to a theatre, or when family members complain about your apathy and indifference to family outings and celebrations. Lack of energy is usually coupled with lack of interest and lack of motivation.

Many patients are loath to admit that their vitality and personality changes may have altered their relationships with their family, friends and work colleagues. For this reason I also encourage patients' partners to sit in during the initial consultation. It is not unusual to hear of quite a different pattern to a patient's behaviour, mood changes and activities from their husband or wife. I am often reminded of my wife's comments on the behavioural and personality differences she had observed in children when she was a teacher. She often needed to point out to concerned parents that, although their child might be 'perfect at home', he/she could be quite different at school.

Unlike many health problems, CFS rarely shows a typical symptom picture. In my experience every patient presents his/her own set of symptoms, which are unique to that person in terms of duration, severity and variety. It is therefore not too surprising that past attempts to offer a widely acceptable definition for CFS have left the medical world with a confusing list of possible titles.

Many doctors and researchers are concerned that including the word 'fatigue' in an official medical term for what can be a very severe condition tends to trivialise it, arguing that no disorder in medicine is named after a single symptom. Also, fatigue is a common feature of a huge range of serious health problems, including heart disease, multiple sclerosis, dementia, respiratory disorders, cancer and many others.

The controversy over a standard description for CFS has led to many options being suggested. These include:

Chronic fatigue and immune dysfunction syndrome (CFIDS)
Chronic immune dysfunctional syndrome (CIDS)
Myalgic encephalomyelitis (ME)
Chronic post-viral fatigue syndrome (CPVFS)
Fibromyalgia syndrome (FBS)
Royal Free disease
Epidemic neurasthenia

You can perhaps understand why I tend to use the term chronic fatigue syndrome (CFS) to describe severe, long-term exhaustion, irrespective of the cause or causes. The title is unambiguous and clear. The selection of a commonly accepted standard term to describe CFS in orthodox medicine remains confusing and controversial, but there is a pattern that is common to all the disorders just listed – undiagnosed severe fatigue. All CFS patients suffer from this while their accompanying symptom complex can vary from patient to patient.

Review of suggested labels for CFS-related conditions
To emphasise the apparent inability for mainstream world medicine to decide on a definitive title for CFS, I list below alternative titles that have been agreed by different countries.

United Kingdom	Royal Free disease
	Post-viral fatigue syndrome (PVFS)
	Yuppie 'flu
	Myalgic encephalomyelitis (ME)
United States of America	Chronic fatigue and immune dysfunction syndrome (CFIDS)
	Chronic fatigue syndrome (CFS)

                           Epidemic neurasthenia
                           Chronic fibromyalgia syndrome (CFS)
                           Immune dysfunction syndrome
New Zealand   Tapanui 'flu
Australia   Chronic fatigue syndrome (CFS)
                           Myalgic encephalomyelitis (ME)

Myalgic encephalomyelitis (ME)

This complicated label – meaning inflammation of the nervous system – highlights a fondness for inventing and using unpronounceable and difficult to spell titles for medical conditions. ME has been defined by the World Health Organisation (WHO) as a 'disease of the nervous system' (*International Classification of Diseases*, No 10, ref. G93.3).

The name ME first appeared in an article in the *Lancet* in 1956. This medical journal reported on an outbreak of sudden fatigue in the Royal Free Hospital in London. At the time many diagnosed this as an example of mass hysteria, and 'Royal Free disease' was added to the list of CFS titles. This fatigue was also thought to have a post-infectious component (post-viral fatigue). Previous outbreaks of fatigue following infections had been reported as far back as the 18th century. Examples of post-infectious symptoms are also associated with glandular fever, Legionnaire's disease, toxoplasmosis (an infection caused by an animal parasite) and the controversial Gulf War syndrome.

The diagnostic criteria for ME and CFS have been defined and listed in many countries. Unfortunately, the lists are not standardised. In fact, they vary with each country. This lack of uniformity in diagnosing and also defining CFS partly explains the confusion this problem is causing within the medical profession.

Diagnostic criteria for CFS and ME in the UK

In the UK the diagnostic criteria for CFS and ME are as follows:

1. A syndrome characterised by fatigue as the principal symptom
2. A syndrome of definite onset that is not lifelong
3. The fatigue is severe, disabling and affects physical and mental functioning

4. The symptom of fatigue should have been present for a minimum of six months, during which time it should have been present for more than 50% of the time

5. Other symptoms may be present, particularly myalgia (muscle pain), mood and sleep disturbance

6. Certain patients should be excluded from this definition, including:
   a. Those with established medical conditions known to produce chronic fatigue (such as severe anaemia). Such patients should be excluded whether the medical condition is diagnosed at presentation or only subsequently. All patients should have a history and physical examination performed by a competent physician.
   b. Those with a current diagnosis of schizophrenia, manic depressive illness, substance abuse, eating disorders or proven organic brain disease. Other psychiatric disorders (including depressive illness, anxiety disorders and hyperventilation syndrome) are not necessarily reasons for exclusion.

Diagnostic criteria for CFS and ME in the USA

In the USA, the diagnostic criteria for CFS, determined by the Centers for Disease Control and Prevention, are:

1. Clinically evaluated, unexplained, persistent or relapsing chronic fatigue that is of new or definite onset (has not been lifelong); is not the result of ongoing exertion; is not substantially relieved by rest; and results in substantial reduction in previous levels of occupational, educational, social or personal activities

2. The concurrent occurrence of *four or more* of the following symptoms, all of which must have persisted or recurred during six or more consecutive months of illness and must not have predated the fatigue:
   a. Self-reported impairment in short-term memory or concentration, severe enough to cause a substantial reduction in previous levels of occupational, educational, social or personal activities
   b. Sore throat
   c. Tender cervical or axillary lymph nodes
   d. Muscle pain

  e. Headaches of a new type, pattern or severity
  f. Unrefreshing sleep
  g. Post-exertional malaise lasting more than 24 hours
  h. Multi joint pain without joint swelling or redness.

Diagnostic criteria for CFS and ME in Australia

In Australia, the diagnostic criteria are:

1. Disabling and prolonged feelings of physical tiredness or fatigue, exacerbated by physical activity
2. Symptoms present for at least six months
3. Unexplained by an alternative diagnosis reached by history, laboratory or physical examinations
4. Accompanied by the new onset of neuropsychological symptoms including impaired short-term memory and concentration, depressed libido and depressed mood. These symptoms usually have their onset at the same time as the physical fatigue, but are typically less severe and less persistent than those seen in classic depressive illness
5. Patients are excluded if:
  a. They have a chronic medical condition that may result in fatigue
  b. There is a history of schizophrenia, other psychotic illnesses or bipolar affective disorder
  c. In addition, drug or alcohol dependence makes CFS very unlikely as a possible diagnosis.

These different requirements for diagnosing CFS make it all too obvious why the medical profession is confused over how to diagnose and treat this increasingly widespread disorder. The main area of disagreement among physicians and researchers is the question, 'What is the central cause of CFS? Is it viral, biochemical, hormonal or psychological, or perhaps a combination of two or more factors?' I shall discuss all these areas in detail, with alternative diagnostic options, in later chapters.

Fibromyalgia syndrome (FMS)

In the early 1840s FMS was defined as 'rheumatism with localised painful areas'. Dr William Gowers (London), in the 1900s, labelled the pain and severe fatigue as 'fibrositis'. In medicine the suffix 'itis' denotes inflammation so fibrositis was therefore not an accurate definition of FMS but purely on one aspect of it. However, in the 1980s the term 'fibromyalgia', which is defined as 'pain in fibres and muscles', replaced both 'fibrositis' and 'rheumatism'.

In 1993 the World Health Organisation (WHO) officially decided that FMS was indeed a syndrome. It was subsequently described as, 'the most common cause of long-term muscle pain coupled with fatigue'. Perhaps a more simple description would be 'fatigue with pain'.

I do occasionally see patients who are fatigued and pain-free but they are a rarity. CFS patients usually complain of muscle and joint stiffness and pain. Characteristically, the symptoms get worse with rest and improve with gentle paced activities. This is the reverse of what happens with many forms of arthritis (rheumatoid arthritis, osteo-arthritis, etc): where inflammation is present, the symptoms get worse during or following exercise and get better with rest.

FMS is now seen as a more complex problem than was previously considered. While pain and fatigue are the dominant symptoms, as many as 30 additional symptoms have been identified as being part of the syndrome. When the WHO defined FMS as a syndrome in 1993 the 'symptom complex' was listed as follows: 'FMS is part of a wider syndrome encompassing headaches, irritable bladder, dysmenorrhoea (period pain), cold sensitivity, Raynaud's disease (poor circulation in fingers and toes, usually in response to cold or stress), restless legs, a typical pattern of numbness and tingling, exercise intolerance and general weakness.'

There exists a galaxy of symptoms within FMS, the commonest being fatigue, depression and poor short-term memory and concentration. A characteristic set of symptoms can also include an unusual heightened sensitivity to light, sound and odour. As with ME and PVF (post-viral fatigue), no single diagnostic test exists to identify the cause or causes of FMS.

Myofascial pain syndrome (MPS)

In common with many disorders that can be seen as CFS-related, MPS is a subject of controversy among many of the researchers and doctors who attempt to diagnose and treat the problem. Although MPS is under the FMS umbrella and frequently seen as part of the CFS group of problems, it does have its own characteristics in terms of causes and symptoms.

MPS and FMS have been termed the 'terrible twosome' (see Dr Chris Jenner's book *Fibromyalgia and Myofascial Pain*). Although the symptoms of MPS are in many ways identical to those of FMS, there is one major difference. Patients with MPS do not usually suffer chronic fatigue. They do, however, experience some secondary fatigue as a result of their insomnia, which is usually caused by their nocturnal pain. Diagnostic confusion exists between FMS and MPS, largely because of their similar symptom patterns and the common tender 'trigger points' that can exist in both conditions. (These trigger points are tender places and were defined in the 1840s as 'tender hard places'.) It seems very likely that these two problems are closely related and, to make exact diagnosis more difficult, many patients suffer from both conditions.

Some practitioners see MPS as a prelude to FMS. The insomnia and night time pain associated with MPS can cause anxiety, depression and fatigue. A vicious circle of pain and fatigue, so characteristic of FMS, can develop as a result of MPS.

The chief symptoms of MPS are:

Common symptoms

1. Muscular stiffness, often with associated joint stiffness
2. Extremity paraesthesia (pins and needles) and numbness
3. Muscular weakness
4. Popping and/or clicking in joints
5. Jaw stiffness
6. Involuntary muscular twitching
7. Trembling in the limbs, often when they are about to be used
8. Insomnia

Less common symptoms

1. Headaches and migraines
2. Poor balance and occasional dizziness
3. Jaw pain and pain in the ears with tinnitus
4. Poor short-term memory and concentration
5. Occasional nausea

6. Intermittent fatigue
7. Anxiety and depression.

Causes of MPS

The most commonly seen causes of MPS offer useful clues to assist in diagnosing the problem. Although, as with FMS, the causes of MPS are subject to considerable debate, the following are widely accepted as the principal reasons for the onset of the symptoms:

1. Accidents, in particular road traffic accidents with whip-lash injuries
2. Falls and various injuries
3. Repetitive strain injuries (usually work based)
4. Stress
5. Hypothyroidism
6. Nutritional deficiencies, such as vitamin D, magnesium, iron and potassium
7. Poor posture and spinal lesions
8. TMJD problems (temporomandibular joint disorder); these can be a result of injury, a misaligned 'bite', upper cervical spinal lesions, etc
9. Viral infections, such as glandular fever.

Dentists not surprisingly have a particular interest in the diagnosis and treatment of MPS as they frequently need to treat misaligned jaws resulting from injury, missing teeth and other causes. Many doctors and dentists hold the view that MPS begins in the jaw and neck.

Studies investigating the relationship between the pain experienced in FMS and the 'trigger' pain points seen in MPS (of which more, later) have shown that up to 70% of the patients studied suffered from both conditions.

Emma's story

Although the causes, diagnosis and treatments for chronic fatigue syndrome are reviewed in detail in later chapters, I have chosen this point to include the first of the case histories in this book that serve to highlight various aspects of the CFS story. Not least, they show the enormous variety of symptoms frequently experienced. The case histories all describe genuine patients with genuine health problems – only names have been changed to ensure patient confidentiality.

I have included Emma's story so early in the book to offer an illustration of the diagnostic and treatment flaws in orthodox medicine, so frequently encountered by the exhausted patients who consult me. The current obsession with 'name dropping' for sets of symptoms, and the medical tendency to diagnose and treat medical conditions and test results, rather than people, is shown in this case history.

Emma had been fatigued since the onset of puberty when she was 12 years of age. When she consulted me she was aged 52 years. Her various intermittent but persistent symptoms had therefore been with her for 40 years. From the age of five years she had suffered from frequent sore throats and earaches, which were treated with numerous courses of antibiotics. Unfortunately, the throat infections persisted and at the age of 12 years, Emma developed convulsions and was given a diagnosis of epilepsy. The convulsions were treated with phenobarbitone for more than two years. Phenobarbitone is a drug regularly prescribed for epilepsy. Unfortunately it has the potential to cause a long list of side-effects. These can include depression, impaired memory, drowsiness, allergic skin reactions and many more. For Emma, the main side-effects were fatigue and weight increase. At 12 years she weighed a little over 12 stone. Her immune system continued to be stressed and antibiotics were still being regularly prescribed for her throat infections.

At the age of 22 years, she developed a kidney infection for which a 'cocktail' of three different antibiotics was prescribed. Shortly after this, Sjögren's syndrome (see Glossary) and rheumatoid arthritis were diagnosed, for which various drugs were tried without much success. These two conditions are classed as auto-immune problems, possibly resulting from Emma's stressed immune system.

A stay in hospital for dental extractions required a general anaesthetic. Emma reacted to the anaesthetic with nausea, which extended her stay in hospital. Reacting to general anaesthetic gas (nitrous oxide) is not unusual.

Disillusioned and depressed, she sought nutritional advice from a complementary practitioner and subsequently, following advice on diet and supplement use, she experienced a general improvement in her health.

In her late 20s, her weight had climbed to 13.7 stone as she had neglected to follow her prescribed diet. Her health again broke down. The Sjögren's syndrome returned, even worse than with her first episode. Ulcers on her eyes were diagnosed, not helped by an allergy to the artificial tears that were prescribed for the dry eyes so characteristics of Sjögren's.

Emma's poor health continued when she developed chronic hiatus hernia in her 30s, which continued to cause symptoms for many years. Gall stones were diagnosed when she was 46 years old, and she had surgery to remove her gall bladder. The anaesthetic again caused severe vomiting for three days, coupled with vertigo. The vertigo was subsequently diagnosed as Ménière's syndrome, but the various drugs prescribed had very little real effect on the symptoms.

In her own words, Emma became an 'anxious recluse'. Her symptoms for over 40 years had included fatigue, severe vertigo, dry skin, hair loss, depression, almost constant nausea, vitiligo and Raynaud's disease. This brings her story up to date with her visit to me, following a practitioner advising her to read my book *Why Am I So Tired?*, which describes an alternative approach to hypothyroidism. Her symptoms also included poor memory and concentration, constipation and general stiffness. The fatigue was worse on rising and better in the afternoon, but worse with delayed or missed meals. An additional cause of concern was a recent diagnosis of SLE (systemic lupus erythematosus), yet another auto-immune condition. Emma also had low blood levels of vitamin B-12 and ferritin (iron reserves) but her GP had not thought treatment was necessary.

In my experience, chronic fatigue very rarely results from a single cause. Emma's health history demonstrated this concept very clearly. Although her diagnosis over the previous 40-plus years had included at least a dozen different health problems, she continued to experience many symptoms, the true causes of which remained undiagnosed and untreated.

Naturopaths often claim that they do not treat diseases; they treat people. I believe that an essential first step in diagnosing any health problem is to identify and treat the more obvious disorders that a patient may be suffering from, including diabetes, anaemia, thyroid problems, high blood pressure, obesity and many other frequently seen and relatively easy to diagnose disorders, but to keep an open mind about what else might be going on.

I am perhaps fortunate in that I am very rarely the first practitioner consulted by my CFS patients. They often initially visit their GP, or perhaps a medical consultant; this results in a variety of laboratory tests, leading to a medical diagnosis and treatment being advised for the common problems listed above. A recent survey I conducted, covering 1000 of my CFS patients, showed that the average duration of their symptoms prior to seeing me was two and a half years. It is therefore not too surprising that the more commonly seen causes of fatigue have very often been identified and treated before I see them.

Although Emma's case history is not presented in the context of any particular underlying problem (unlike the case histories in chapter 6), I hope that it serves to show readers the complexity of CFS symptoms and diagnosis, and emphasises the misdiagnosis that is so prevalent in medical practice – a situation that current NHS protocols, coupled with restraints on GPs' time with patients, is failing to improve. Given Emma's medical history you may well be asking:

1. After so many years of diagnosis and treatment, why was Emma still exhausted and ill?
2. Just what did you as a naturopath advise her to do to complement, or replace, the drugs and treatment already prescribed?

My answers to these questions serve to highlight the differences between orthodox and alternative approaches to CFS. This comparison demonstrates why naturopathic treatment was eventually more successful for Emma than the painkillers, antibiotics, antacids, anti-depressants, tonics, anti-inflammatories, insomnia drugs, artificial tears and surgery that had been prescribed for her over many years for over a dozen different health problems. This provides a foretaste of my approach throughout this book and describes how naturopaths work.

The initial challenge that presents with any case history as complex as Emma's is to identify and separate symptoms and causes. The other important priority is to attempt to match patients' test results with their symptoms. Such matching can be very reassuring to someone who has never been offered a satisfactory diagnosis. I see so many patients who have been informed that, as their blood tests do not show abnormal readings, their fatigue must be caused by depression, insomnia, anxiety and probably too much stress.

Chapter 1

It was clear to me that Emma's central problem from an early age had been the breakdown of her immune system, beginning with throat infections at five years of age. Many factors have the potential to adversely influence our immune function. One effect of this is auto-immune diseases – a large group of diseases that result from our immune system attacking our own body. There are many doctors and researchers who believe that the majority of human illnesses are a result of immune system breakdown. The conditions that are included under the auto-immune disease heading include rheumatoid arthritis, Crohn's disease, ulcerative colitis, multiple sclerosis, thyroiditis, lupus, scleroderma (SLE), adrenal fatigue, diabetes (type I), pernicious anaemia (B-12 deficiency), Sjögren's syndrome, Raynaud's phenomenon and polycystic ovary syndrome (PCOS).

The usual medical treatment is to prescribe drugs to suppress what is seen as an overactive or misdirected immune system. These drugs include antibiotics, steroids and pain killers. An unfortunate and frequently seen result of such treatment is a further weakening of a patient's immunity, leading to more serious infections. This is usually coupled with adrenal hormone deficiencies and resulting inflammation in various tissues and organs. Emma's history included several auto-immune conditions, including lupus, B-12 deficiency, rheumatoid arthritis and Sjögren's and Raynaud's syndromes, which had all been treated with drugs designed to suppress her immune system and offer transient symptom relief.

Although fatigue is a commonly experienced symptom in auto-immune disorders, I considered that Emma's current fatigue was principally a result of four disorders that had never been satisfactorily addressed by her doctors – namely, her underactive thyroid, her adrenal fatigue with resulting symptoms of hypoglycaemia (low blood sugar), and her low levels of blood ferritin (iron reserves) and vitamin B-12.

Although Emma had been tested for thyroid hormones, ferritin and vitamin B-12 on several occasions, no action had been taken as the results were not considered sufficiently abnormal to warrant treatment, all the results being at the lower end of the 'normal' ranges. The medical establishment's slavish fixation with normal ranges for diagnosis, irrespective of a patient's age, symptoms or health history, is a topic that I shall return to frequently throughout this book.

However, to return to Emma, I requested my 'fatigue blood profile' (see chapter 5, page 107), which includes thyroid function, blood ferritin and vitamin B-12 levels. Although I regularly use five laboratories for testing, I send the majority of my patients to the Doctors Laboratory in central London. The results were as follows:

Free T4 (thyroxine)	13.8 pmol/l	Normal range: 12–22 pmol/l
Ferritin (iron reserves)	18 µg/l	Normal range: 12–150 µg/l
Vitamin B-12	185 pg/ml	Normal range: 190–600 pg/ml

As you can see, Emma's results were all 'sub-clinical', a term which is defined as, 'An illness that stays below the surface of clinical detection. A subclinical disease therefore has no recognisable clinical findings, being distinct from a "clinical" disease which has signs and symptoms that can be recognised.'

The usual clinical findings when investigating fatigue are blood test results. Emma's doctors' responses to her sub-clinical results highlight the principal flaw in the medical diagnosis of CFS – test results are analysed in isolation and not as part of a whole clinical picture. I believe that the appropriate test results *must* be interpreted with direct reference to the patient's symptoms, This is the essential first step in understanding the causes of their CFS, and devising subsequent effective treatment strategies. (With regard to choosing appropriate tests, I shall outline the importance of blood test selection and interpretation in later chapters.)

All the results of Emma's three tests were borderline. Meanwhile, her vitality and stamina were undoubtedly compromised, presumably by her borderline hypothyroidism and low iron and vitamin B-12 levels.

I requested one further test – an 'adrenal stress profile'. This involves measuring the adrenal hormones cortisol and DHEA (that is, 'dehydroepiandrosterone', which for obvious reasons is usually referred to as DHEA) in a patient's saliva four times over a 24-hour period. The adrenal test confirmed my suspicions, as Emma's results showed 'adrenal fatigue', with both hormones being too low. (It is not unusual for both the adrenal and thyroid glands to be under-functioning. The thyroid gland tends to reflect our metabolic rate and is therefore often depressed with anaemia also.)

I always ask my patients to give me details of a typical three-day diet. This should include *all* food and drink and the timing of meals. Emma's diet was not ideal. She usually missed breakfast, favoured sugar-rich snacks and coffees and avoided red meat. A radical change would be needed.

Emma's treatment programme

With the test results, health history and diet details, I was able to design a treatment programme for Emma, the basic components of which were as follows.

Diet

I advised radical changes. Emma needed to eat red meat at least twice weekly, including offal, with a preference for lamb or beef. Also fish twice weekly. As it seemed likely that Emma's frequent episodes of low blood sugar were contributing to her current symptoms, I gave her a copy of my low blood sugar diet. This is described in full in chapter 6 (see page 149) but in summary comprises the following guidelines:

> Avoid sugar, sugar-rich foods and carbohydrates
> Avoid soft drinks, caffeine, chocolate, alcohol and tobacco
> Eat an early, protein-rich breakfast and a late supper
> Eat four meals daily, each with a protein component.

Such a regime would help to stabilise her blood sugar levels, and reduce the strain on her fatigued adrenal system, thereby providing refreshing sleep and more vitality on rising.

Emma's supplement programme

Emma's health problems were neither trivial nor short term. It was therefore essential that that she should take specific nutritional supplements to balance her metabolism, improve her mental and physical energy and protect her over-stressed immune system. Simply advising an over-the-counter vitamin/mineral supplement was not going to work. The lists that follow include supplements the ingredients of which are described in the Glossary at the end of the book (see page 253).

Objective 1 – Immune system support

Cell protection from free-radical damage was needed. Free radical sources include air pollution, cigarette smoke, stress (physical and emotional) and excessive exercise. This protection is provided by anti-oxidants which I advised Emma to take. These included:

Co-enzyme Q-10	N-acetyl cysteine	Vitamin A
Glutathione	Omega-3 fatty acids	Vitamin C
Grape seed extract	Quercetin	Vitamin E

Fortunately, many of these antioxidant nutrients are included in combined formulas. Nutri supply 'Plant Source Antioxidants', and Biovea supply their 'Anti-oxidant Formula'. Taking a formula serves to reduce the number of tablets taken each day.

Objective 2 – Increase thyroid and adrenal function

With the deficiencies shown in Emma's test results, thyroid and adrenal glandulars were essential supplements for her. I also recommended 'Thyro-Complex' which I designed for Nutri and GTF complex, which provides nutrients to treat low blood sugar. In total I therefore prescribed the following:

GTF Complex	Nutri Adrenal Extra	Nutri Thyroid
Thyro Complex		

Objective 3 – Improve vitamin B-12 and iron deficiencies

I prescribed vitamin B-12 injections twice weekly and advised Emma to take additional B-12 as capsules each day that included the intrinsic factor to assist B-12 absorption. I also recommended chelated iron tablets. In these, the iron is bound to protein to facilitate easy absorption.

The schedule was as follows:

Vitamin B-12 (1 mg) injections twice weekly
Intrinsic B-12/folate twice daily
Hemagenics – easily absorbed iron taken twice daily.

Objective 4 – Treatment with supplements to reduce anxiety and depression

Although Emma's state of mind evidently resulted from her poor health, it was also essential to reduce her anxiety and give her some symptom relief. I therefore recommended the following supplements:

- GABA (Gamma-amino butyric acid) – has been defined as 'nature's valium', and the 'perfect tranquiliser'; it is a neurotransmitter, the lack of which can cause depression and anxiety; also seizures in children.
- 5-HTP (5-Hydroxytryptophan) – a natural plant-sourced precursor of the neurotransmitter serotonin; it is a mood enhancer and a useful sleep-aid.
- Probiotics every day to replenish beneficial gut bacteria.

This complex programme produced an improvement in Emma's symptoms after three months. Further blood tests and adrenal saliva tests confirmed that her ferritin, vitamin B-12, thyroid and adrenal function were all around 25% increased. With such a long-term history of ill health, it would be 12–18 months before Emma was fully recovered.

In conclusion

The central difficulty when attempting to define CFS and give it a universally acceptable title is the double problem of severity and duration. There is also the confusion surrounding other symptoms that usually accompany the chronic fatigue; hence its full title, 'chronic fatigue syndrome' where 'syndrome' means a collection of symptoms that tend to occur together.

The various diagnostic criteria offered by different countries provide credibility for CFS as a medical condition, but there still remains a public and medical resistance to using the term chronic fatigue syndrome to describe the status of exhausted patients.

Symptom severity is difficult to determine. Most of us recognise that a typical headache can be demonstrably very different in severity when compared with a migraine that requires the sufferer to retreat to bed in a darkened room for two to three days, particularly if the migraine is accompanied by frequent vomiting and near blindness. Regrettably, fatigue severity is not so easy to establish.

I believe that the variety of definitions offered to explain CFS over the previous 40 to 50 years, and the range of names used for the condition, have contributed to the confusion. For this reason, and also to reassure exhausted patients that their symptoms are not imaginary, I prefer to call the condition chronic fatigue syndrome, or CFS, and shall do so throughout this book.

I shall conclude this chapter with a quotation from the front page of the *Daily Telegraph* (4 October 2012). The article was entitled, 'Doctors regard patients as conditions not people'. It went on to say, 'Patients suffer poor care in NHS hospitals because they are viewed by doctors and nurses as "medical conditions" to deal with, instead of people, the Royal College of Physicians warns today.' It is significant that this criticism was not made by the alternative medicine lobby, but from within the medical establishment itself.

Chapter 2

The symptoms of chronic fatigue syndrome

In this chapter I will describe the typical symptoms of chronic fatigue syndrome (CFS). I will discuss the diagnosis and causes in later chapters, together with medical and non-medical treatment options.

Those readers who are victims of severe and often disabling exhaustion may wonder why a chapter that describes the symptoms of CFS is really necessary. Many consider that fatigue is a level of tiredness, an easily recognised and frequently experienced symptom – a symptom that we have all encountered, at some time in our lives, and become familiar with. There are those who view CFS as simply a more severe version of everyday tiredness. Unfortunately, there is a general tendency for the public and for GPs to underestimate the severity and the variety of the symptoms that are so often part of CFS.

When I have discussed this attitude with many of my CFS patients, it has become clear that they are distressed at the apparent lack of understanding shown by their families, friends, employers and doctors. Frequently expressed responses to those suffering severe long-term exhaustion can include: 'You need a good holiday'; 'Try to get more sleep'; 'Learn to relax'; 'Take up a hobby'; 'Get some anti-depressants'; 'We all get tired; don't work so hard'. Such hurtful and pointless comments draw attention to the commonly held view that CFS is a personality or life-style problem and therefore not really an illness, the implication being that it can only be solved by the sufferer's own efforts. This seems a very good reason to outline the vast number of symptoms that can be included in the condition.

When I meet patients for their initial consultation, I always allow at least 60 minutes to discuss their previous health history, family history, lifestyle and diet, current and previous diagnosis and treatment. However, much of the time is generally given over to the description of their current symptoms, these after all being the chief reason for their appointment.

The variety of symptoms in CFS can often exceed 20 and is rarely less than 10. Such a large range can cause many patients to be frustrated by the current trend in UK general practices to deliberately limit patients' symptom discussions to two to three per visit.

One of the most distressing and annoying symptoms that people with CFS suffer is confusion and poor short-term memory. It is not unusual to hear them quite accurately describe memories of their childhood in some detail, yet forget where they have left their mobile phone or where they have parked their car. For this reason, I make use of a 'tick-off' symptom questionnaire list to refresh their memory and to provide a comprehensive picture of their physical and mental problems.

Symptoms have been described as the body's many cries for help, or as 'diagnostic clues'. Even trivial symptoms that a patient may be too embarrassed, or forgetful, to mention can sometimes provide very useful aids to diagnosis. This means it is important to include problems you may regard as trivial when you see your doctor/health practitioner.

CFS – the symptoms

It needs to be emphasised that there is no 'typical' symptom-picture with CFS. Even the commonest symptom – fatigue – is variable and subject to many different patterns and interpretations. It is estimated that approximately 25% of patients visiting their GP complain that they are 'tired all the time'. Fatigue is a symptom, not a sign – that is, it is something the patient experiences (subjective) and has to tell the practitioner about, while 'signs' are clues the practitioner can spot for him/herself and generally measure (objective). For example, a patient may *look* tired and pale, with a stressed facial expression and a slumped posture (all 'signs'), but cosmetics and a forced cheerfulness can quite often disguise an exhausted patient.

Chapter 2

Fatigue

The fatigue that results from many health problems – including, for example, anaemia, insomnia, depression, arthritis and infections, in addition to major illnesses – usually follows a pattern. It will generally begin gradually, improve with rest and be worse at the end of the day. The fatigue of CFS has quite a different paradigm. I have yet to talk to a CFS patient who claims to be better on rising and worse at the end of the day. A frequent question that patients ask is, 'Why do I feel so tired when I awaken but have spare vitality in the evening?' In people who do not suffer from un-refreshing sleep, or severe and long-term insomnia, the morning lethargy, both mental and physical, seems illogical and confusing.

The commonest disorder causing chronic tiredness is iron-deficient anaemia (see chapter 3 on causes, page 41). With this problem a patient usually feels a little more vital after a night's sleep but his/her energy gradually fades throughout the day. With CFS, available energy can vary before and after meals, with different foods, and, in women, vitality may flag before the start of periods. Spare stamina is always in short supply and recovery from stress and infections can be unnaturally slow.

Surprisingly, the fatigue of CFS can start quite suddenly. There is rarely a gradual symptom build-up. Patients can often pinpoint their symptom onset to a particular, memorable day. Suspected 'trigger' factors can include any of the following:

> A road traffic accident, particularly involving a whip-lash injury or blow to the head
> Dental work with mercury amalgam removal
> Infections, notably 'flu or glandular fever
> Foreign travel, particularly including Asia and the Far East
> Severe stress from, for example, a divorce, a house move, child birth, change of job etc
> Surgery with a general anaesthetic
> Drug side-effects.

The expression often used about these triggers is, 'the proverbial last straw'. I shall explain later (see chapter 4, page 74) in more detail just how and why these triggers can set off CFS.

Pain and stiffness

Pain is our commonest symptom. We tend to associate pain and stiffness with damage or disease, but they can also be common symptoms of many functional health problems that cannot be identified in scans, x-rays or tests. Examples include headaches, neuralgias, cramp, numbness, indigestion and many other symptoms. One such condition that seems to defy a standard diagnosis is 'fibromyalgia' (FMS), once termed 'fibrositis' or 'rheumatism'. It is very rare for CFS sufferers to be free from muscle and joint stiffness and pain.

As with fatigue, such symptoms usually get worse with rest, particularly on rising, and improve with gentle activity.

Specific pain trigger areas can often be 'mapped' in fibromyalgia patients.

Poor memory and concentration

We tend to think of memory loss as a symptom of getting old in general, and of dementia and Alzheimer's disease in particular. The memory loss experienced by CFS patients is quite different. I have found that exhausted patients of all ages can experience this symptom – the young as much as the old – and a characteristic with CFS patients is that it is the recent and short-term memory that usually falters, with the sufferer being fully aware of the problem. (The loss of memory that goes with dementia does not involve this same self-awareness.) Their capacity to recall long-past events, names and people is often intact. Typical examples would be forgetting the day or date; forgetting to collect children from school, to feed the dog, to do the shopping, or to telephone a friend; missing birthdays and anniversaries; forgetting food in the oven and the location of car keys or their handbag. There can be a long and embarrassing list of things forgotten; this has been termed 'the handbag in the fridge syndrome', for obvious reasons.

Poor memory and concentration are closely linked symptoms. Lapses in concentration, or 'brain fog', are very typical of CFS, so much so that I always give my patients written and detailed memos or instructions, never trusting to verbal advice.

For those who suffer from CFS, books cease to be a pleasure, as plots and names cannot be remembered. The modern trend to include a character list in certain books can be a great help. In this book, I have repeated a certain amount of information so that readers with CFS do not have to hold too much in their memories to understand new points that I am making.

Crossword puzzles and computer games are not always completed. Conversations can be an effort and social activities are usually reduced. How often do many people like to start a conversation with, 'Do you remember...?' Thinking requires energy; the brain needs fuel to function efficiently and thinking is a chemical process. It is therefore not too surprising that one's memory and concentration are adversely influenced in CFS. Physical and mental exhaustion are usually parallel symptoms. Those of us who are physically exhausted are rarely mentally alert. The former US President Bill Clinton, who claimed to need only five hours sleep each night, once admitted, 'Every important mistake I've made in my life, I've made because I was too tired'.

Depression

In mainstream medicine, depression is thought to be the root course of many symptoms and health problems. Certainly fatigue is often top of the list of symptoms said to be caused by depression. It must be very tempting and time-saving for a general practitioner to say, 'You are tired because you are depressed' as this diagnosis is usually followed by a prescription for anti-depressants. The doctor can then feel that something has been done to help.

In my experience, CFS patients do not feel any more vital when taking anti-depressants. I believe this is because the fatigue causes the depression and not the other way around. I have seen this view confirmed many times when a patient's depression lifts as his/her vitality improves. A tired body causes a tired mind, and physical and mental exhaustion are partners.

Anxiety

Anxiety is another very common symptom of CFS. Readers will probably not be surprised at this. I have spoken to CFS patients who have been out of work for a year or more. Their libido is often non-existent; frequently they are separated from their partner. Many are wheelchair bound and quite unable to be out of their beds for more than three to four hours each day. They have often lost contact with friends, family and neighbours, so it would be very strange if they did not suffer from anxiety. Unfortunately, as I shall describe elsewhere in this book (see page 56), anxiety and depression can be a contributing causes of fatigue. Hence a vicious circle can be established as follows:

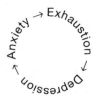

This is a commonly seen feature of CFS. Regrettably, anxiety and depression are often confused in people's minds with worry and unhappiness. This results in the frequently heard advice to CFS patients who are suspected of malingering to 'pull yourself together'. The GP's definition, *plumbum oscillans* ('swinging the lead'), is a frequently seen diagnosis written on a patient's case notes. These symptoms represent an area of diagnosis where assessment of symptom duration and severity can be critically important in establishing a diagnosis and treatment strategy. To tell an exhausted, desperate patient that his/her symptoms are 'all in the mind' can be both insulting and unproductive.

Circulation symptoms

Changes in blood flow can influence many symptoms that are commonly included in the CFS 'menu'. Perhaps the most obvious is the efficiency of the body's thermostat. CFS patients complain of 'always feeling cold', yet night sweats and hot flushes are quite common. The following symptoms may also be influenced by inappropriate changes in blood supply:

Paraesthesia of hands and feet (pins and needles)
Numbness in extremities (fingers and toes)
Muscle cramping
Restless legs – chiefly at night
Bruising without any apparent cause
Heart palpitations
Sensitivity to weather changes and temperature

Poor and slow wound healing

Low blood pressure (hypotension) – this can be experienced as loss of balance with dizziness when changing position ('postural hypotension')

Headaches – often severe, with visual symptoms and nausea, as often experienced with migraine; such symptoms are often worse on rising and before the start of periods.

Immune system symptoms

Stress is a common component of CFS, and stress depresses and weakens the efficiency of our immune system. Many symptoms of CFS can provide clues to suggest that a patient's immune system is struggling. Many world-class athletes suffer from repeated infections, as a result of the adrenal exhaustion that can result from their intense training and competing.

Some of the symptoms that are linked to a weakened immune system include:

Auto-immune conditions

Frequent sore throats

Lymph node swelling and pain, in the neck and under the arms

Rashes linked to shingles

Chronic coughing with chest pain

Dyspnoea (shortness of breath)

Frequent infections with slow recovery

A low body temperature, coupled with being frequently feverish – especially at night

Poor healing of cuts, abrasions and bruises

Candidiasis, thrush or yeast sensitivity, with cystitis.

Hormonal (endocrine) symptoms

Our hormone-producing glands, sometimes referred to as the 'endocrine axis', comprise the hypothalamus, the pituitary gland, the thyroid gland, the adrenal glands and the ovaries or testes. There is plenty of evidence available to confirm the important influence that these glands have on CFS, particularly when they are depressed or fatigued. Up to 50% of CFS patients have a borderline underactive thyroid gland and just as many show signs of adrenal fatigue, with hypoglycaemia (low blood sugar) being a frequent effect.

Fatigue is a feature of many glandular conditions. Other symptoms that are a result of hormonal deficiencies include:

Low blood sugar (hypoglycaemia)
Muscle stiffness and pain (myalgia)
Insomnia
Anxiety
Reduced sex drive (low libido)
Pre-menstrual syndrome (PMS)
Period pain (dysmenorrhoea)
Polycystic ovary syndrome (PCOS)
Heavy periods (menorrhagia)
Hair loss (alopecia)
Dry eyes and mouth (Sjögren's syndrome)
Endometriosis
Increased weight and fluid retention
Mood swings.

Digestive symptoms

I have yet to meet a patient with CFS who can boast an efficient, symptom-free digestive system. Our muscles are rendered less efficient with CFS and the digestive system is largely a muscular system. Gut transit (that is, movement from one part of the gut to the next) becomes irregular and symptoms caused by this can include stomach fullness and wind, alternating constipation and diarrhoea, abdominal pain, colic, nausea and dehydration. Such symptoms are frequently termed 'irritable bowel syndrome'. Problems with gut permeability ('leaky gut') are also common.

Other digestive symptoms seen with CFS include food intolerances; allergic reactions to cosmetics, household products, animals, insects and drugs can contribute to CFS symptoms and digestive symptoms. The development of new reactions is a common feature, and existing sensitivities may get worse.

Less common symptoms

In addition to the symptoms I have listed already, there are many that occur less frequently, but often enough definitely to be associated with CFS (perhaps in 10–15% of patients). These can include the following:

Taste, smell, hearing and vision changes, often with 'photophobia' (intolerance of light)

Disturbed sleep, with nightmares

Epileptic-type seizures, even blackouts

Alcohol intolerance

Coffee and sugar craving

Irritability, usually as a result of delayed meals and on rising

Attention-deficit disorder (ADD)

Histamine reactions, including rhinitis, breathlessness and hives

Discomfort and frequency with urination

Various types of rashes

Carpal tunnel syndrome

Referred pains or neuralgias, such as sciatica, brachial neuritis, facial pain

Bleeding, sensitive gums and tongue

New-found sensitivity to weather changes

Unnatural thirst (such as in dehydration, or diabetes).

After reading this chapter with its catalogue of so many different symptoms, you will not be surprised that those who suffer from CFS are frequently unhappy with their doctor's relative indifference to their poor health. To emphasise the diversity and complexity of the numerous symptoms that CFS patients may suffer, I describe below the symptoms listed by two of my CFS patients, with their permission.

You will appreciate that there are many symptoms of CFS that are unique to female patients, chiefly attributed to female hormone problems, pregnancy and menopause. There are very few symptoms linked to CFS that are unique to males. Not surprisingly then, the balance of female to male patients in my practice is around 12 to one in favour of females. To highlight a few of the differences in symptom patterns between the sexes, I have therefore included symptom lists for a male and a female patient (see box on next page).

Box 2.1

Mary's symptoms	**Tom's symptoms**
Housewife – Aged 42 years	*Solicitor – Aged 54 years*
Chronic, severe fatigue	Chronic fatigue
Poor memory and concentration	Severe migraines with nausea
Pain, in the joints (worse with rest)	Cold extremities
Muscle stiffness (worse in the morning)	Nocturnal cramp
Overweight by 3 stone/18 kg	General muscle stiffness (worse with rest)
Anxious, depressed and irritable	Occasional dizziness with poor balance, worse with changing position
Pre-menstrual syndrome (sugar craving, weight increase and irritability)	Photophobia, with poor focusing
Period pain (dysmenorrhoea)	Fullness and discomfort after meals, with hiatus hernia
Severe nocturnal restless legs	Constipation
Night cramps	Depressed and anxious
Insomnia	Irritable and very sleepy with missed meals
'Always cold'	General lethargy on rising
Bruises easily	Several food allergies, mainly reacting to dairy products
Poor libido	
Stomach fullness after meals, with acid reflux	
Constipation	
Frequent sore throats	
Frequent colds with rhinitis	
Morning headaches	
Sugar cravings after delayed meals	
Chronic vaginal thrush (*Candida albicans*)	

Making sense of symptoms

Although these lists help to demonstrate the great diversity in the symptoms experienced by those who suffer CFS, there is another important variable to be taken into account whenever such symptoms are discussed and assessed. This is the *severity* of symptoms.

Some symptoms can be fairly accurately matched to patients' test results – for example, iron-deficient anaemia. The level of the test results can provide a useful clue to identify the severity of a patient's fatigue. There are, however, many symptoms that cannot be judged or defined simply by reliance on a person's blood test results. By definition, symptoms are subjective and only the patient can experience them. Only he/she can describe the effect of symptoms on his/her physical and mental well-being.

One of the central challenges when a practitioner is consulted by a CFS patient for a diagnosis and possible treatment, is to determine what are the causes and what are the symptoms. As I have said already, chronic fatigue is never the only symptom in CFS. I always send prospective new patients a set of forms to complete prior to the first consultation (our 'New patient pack' – see end of this chapter, pages 36–37). These forms can be likened to a health 'CV', with questions on symptoms, past health, past and current treatment, family history and typical meals over three days. Many useful and relevant facts can thus be made available for me at our first meeting and this information can provide valuable clues to a possible diagnosis. Regrettably, the patient's answers are sometimes superficial and lacking in detail.

By definition, CFS is associated with a long-term set or group of symptoms. For many exhausted and often desperate people, the symptoms that accompany their chronic fatigue have become a familiar part of their life. The relevance of many such symptoms can easily be overlooked or ignored when a practitioner is attempting to diagnose their problems.

What is normal?

When I discuss symptom duration and severity with patients, particularly those who are passing through puberty, teenage years, pregnancy, menopause or past retirement age, I am quite regularly asked, 'Aren't these normal symptoms to be expected at my time of life?' The assumption is that at certain times in one's life, predictable symptoms surface that are normal and inevitable. Sufferers, assuming they are experiencing 'normal' symptoms, do not mention them to any health practitioner and find ways of learning to live with them. Some examples may help to illustrate this. It seems appropriate to begin by looking at children's' symptoms. And yes, I do occasionally see exhausted children as patients.

The 'terrible twos'

There are probably many readers who do not agree that young children can suffer from CFS, yet I do see very young patients with exhaustion and disturbed sleep. Their parents ask that important question: 'Surely many of these symptoms are quite *normal* for two-year-olds?' While there are many two-year-olds who are hyperactive and irritable, with fussy eating habits and disturbed sleep this cannot be put down simply to their age. It is often a consequence of poor quality diets and/or changes in routine and sleeping patterns that can distress children of this age. (Although young children do not usually telephone me for consultations, I often see the mothers of very young children who are exhausted themselves, in part as a result of their child's behaviour.)

Puberty

Puberty (on average nine to 13 years for girls and 10 to 14 years for boys) is another time in life that serves to justify the notion that a whole range of symptoms are *normal* and only to be expected in some children. These symptoms include acne, being overweight, being irritable and argumentative in the early morning and often fatigued. However, there are clearly defined and treatable reasons for such symptoms, which I shall discuss in detail later in the book. A healthy young person should not have to suffer these problems.

Teenagers – 15–20 years+

I am sure that many readers will have observed changes in young people's health when they leave home. So often such changes are simply put down to their being teenagers. I consider that there are well-defined reasons for teenage 'symptoms', such as nutrient-deficient junk food diets, sometimes obsession with weight (as in bulimia and anorexia), and excessive use of caffeine, alcohol, tobacco and recreational drugs, in addition to the unfamiliar stress of new relationships, studies and leaving the family environment. These factors are more likely to affect a teenager's health and vitality than the simple fact of their age.

Pregnancy

Pregnancy is not an illness. Such symptoms as morning sickness, being overweight, mood changes, obsessive food cravings, fatigue and post-natal depression all may have treatable causes. It seems very likely that pregnancy along with puberty, teenage life, menopause and perhaps old age, will in the near future all be officially defined as medical syndromes. Even 'peri-menopause' is becoming an accepted medical term to explain a set of symptoms that can arise 10 years before the usual menopause age. Certainly, pre-menstrual syndrome and post-natal depression are commonly used terms to explain a set of typical female symptoms. Unfortunately, their frequency serves to endorse and define them as near normal.

Menopause

How many women suffering a wide range of distressing symptoms have been 'reassured' by their GP that they need not be too concerned, as they are 'going through the menopause'? This implies that such symptoms are to be expected and are almost certainly a result of temporary and normal female hormone imbalances. The so-called 'symptoms' of menopause can include fatigue, personality changes, libido loss, being overweight, muscle and joint pain, depression and hot flushes. Once again, female patients are encouraged to believe that such symptoms are transient and normal. I have talked to patients in their late 70s and early 80s who continue to experience nightly hot flushes and have never returned to a normal weight, even after discontinuing their periods 20 to 30 years previously. Unfortunately, their post-menopausal fatigue can also persist for many years after menopause.

Post-retirement old age

Why is it that doctors 'allow us to feel exhausted when we are elderly without suffering any specific illness'? We accept that we are not likely to be dynamic at 80 years of age, yet I personally know friends and colleagues in their mid-80s who can put me to shame in any 'vitality' stakes. Old age is not a disease. Allowing for normal wear and tear, unless we are suffering from a major illness, we should have learned to pace ourselves as we age. Eating sensibly and controlling our stress handling (that is, our ability to cope with stress) and life-style sufficiently wisely, should enable us to avoid exhaustion. Yet age is often seen as just another 'normal' explanation for the symptoms of CFS. 'What do you expect at your age?' is a fairly widely heard question asked by medical professionals to patients and also amongst friends, family members and colleagues.

Male or female?

Finally there is one more factor that can cause the symptoms of CFS to be classed as 'normal': gender-bias. It is very probable that women *are* more prone to neurosis, depression and cravings than are men. The links between female hormone status, adrenal function and blood sugar levels serve to explain this gender bias. With many female health problems there are neuro-emotional components – for example, anorexia and bulimia as chiefly seen in teenage girls, 'pre-menstrual syndrome' in women approaching average menopause age, and post-natal depression following childbirth.

Unfortunately, the medical profession seems to hold the view that many of their fatigued female patients between the ages of 40 and 60 are inclined to be neurotic. 'Neurotic' is often a word used as an 'explain all' diagnosis for CFS. I regularly see evidence of this medical opinion when discussing previous prescriptions that have been offered to my exhausted patients. The ratio of anti-depressants prescribed for CFS for females and males is around 10 to one. In fact, I rarely see CFS male patients who have been prescribed an anti-depressant, yet with the female patients, particularly in the 45–55 years age range, such drugs seem to be handed out with the regularity of aspirin or paracetamol. As physical exhaustion and many other distressing symptoms are included under the CFS umbrella, it is not at all surprising that many of such patients are profoundly distressed, anxious and depressed. They receive a prescription for anti-depressants in response to the faulty medical view that many of their symptoms are a result of depression. In fact, depression is just one of the symptoms of CFS and to single out one symptom for treatment is, I believe, on a par with prescribing analgesics as the single remedy for toothache.

After reading this section about 'what is normal', you may assume that I consider a patient's age to be an important component in CFS diagnosis. This is not my view, although a person's age can be a contributing factor. My point is that age-related symptoms, as described above, are so often experienced in modern life that they are assumed to be normal. If they are not included when patients discuss their symptoms, this can lead to many important background causes of CFS being ignored or simply discounted.

Chapter summary

The many symptoms typically suffered by CFS patients could quite easily provide sufficient material for a separate book. More detailed symptom lists are included in the case histories in chapter 6.

This chapter attempts to describe the most commonly experienced symptoms. However, as the syndrome has the potential to influence all our body systems adversely, there are many less common symptoms that can occur with CFS. I have included lists of symptoms for real-life two patients in order to emphasise the great diversity of such symptoms. Although, by definition, fatigue is the dominant symptom seen in CFS, there are many individual variations.

Pre-consultation questionnaire

NAME: D.O.B:

MARITAL STATUS: OCCUPATION:

NAME, ADDRESS AND TELEPHONE NUMBER OF YOUR GP:
(Your GP will NOT be contacted without your consent)

PLEASE INSERT YOUR DAILY QUANTITIES OF THE FOLLOWING:

ALCOHOL…………………….   COFFEE……………… (sugar)…………)

CIGARETTES………………..   TEA………………… (sugar)……..…..)

SOFT DRINKS………………....   CHOCS/SWEETS…………..……………

ARE YOU OR HAVE YOU EVER BEEN A BLOOD DONOR?   YES / NO

CURRENT SYMPTOMS:

PLEASE LIST ANY PRESCRIPTION DRUGS YOU ARE CURRENTLY TAKING:

PLEASE LIST ANY SUPPLEMENTS YOU ARE CURRENTLY TAKING:

A BRIEF MEDICAL HISTORY:

Continue overleaf

3 DAY DIARY (FOOD & DRINK)					
Day 1		Day 2		Day 3	
Time	Breakfast	Time	Breakfast	Time	Breakfast
Time	Snack	Time	Snack	Time	Snack
Time	Lunch	Time	Lunch	Time	Lunch
Time	Snack	Time	Snack	Time	Snack
Time	Dinner	Time	Dinner	Time	Dinner
Time	Snack	Time	Snack	Time	Snack

Chapter 3

The common causes of chronic fatigue syndrome

Throughout this book I have used the term 'chronic fatigue syndrome' (CFS) to describe severe, long-term exhaustion, irrespective of the cause or causes. This allows the term 'CFS' to embrace the many terms that imply a single cause, be they 'post-viral syndrome', 'myalgic encephalomyelitis' or 'immune dysfunction syndrome'. It is also compatible with my experience that most patients' exhaustion is caused by a number of interrelated problems, as I will explain in this chapter.

Does chronic fatigue syndrome have a physical cause?

Ever since 'rapid-onset severe fatigue' was reported in the *Lancet* in 1956 the cause, or causes, of chronic fatigue syndrome (CFS) has/have been a matter of controversy. Is it a purely psychological phenomenon or is there a physical cause? The *Lancet* report described an epidemic of chronic fatigue at London's Royal Free Hospital which affected both staff and a few patients in 1955; it was thought by many to be the result of mass hysteria, but by others to result from a mystery virus. The term 'myalgic encephalomyelitis' (ME) was coined at that time to embrace the assumption that the condition involved inflammation of the central nervous system, with muscle pain. In the USA, the term 'post-viral fatigue syndrome' (PVFS) has since largely replaced 'ME', again implying a viral cause.

A study at Colombia University in New York in 2009 suggested a possible link between certain rare viruses, distantly related to HIV, and CFS. Identifying a proven viral cause for the symptoms of CFS was seen as the Holy Grail in finding the biological explanation for unexplained fatigue. Unfortunately, a report in 2012 cast doubt on the validity of the Columbia testing procedures as new work could find no evidence of a viral link. The same researchers were involved in each of the studies and their latest report has confirmed conclusively that the viral theory was incorrect. Similar studies in London and Holland also failed to show a viral cause for CFS.

These results have tended to back up the majority view of many scientists and doctors that CFS is largely psychological in its cause, and that the exhaustion and pain so characteristic of the condition can be correlated with certain personality traits.

To my mind, this ongoing debate tends to expose the chief flaw in the medical perspective – that there must be one cause to explain CFS. Having treated the condition for over 40 years, I do not accept that there can be one single cause for the huge diversity of symptoms, both physical and mental. Many of the exhausted people who consult me present with a large range of health problems (sometimes as many as eight conditions) that are contributing to their symptoms. It is therefore important to be aware of the range of issues that can contribute to CFS, noting that many of them are interrelated. In this chapter I will describe what I have found to be the most common contributory factors; I will look at the less commonly seen causes in the next chapter. To demonstrate the complexity of CFS causation I have included a series of case histories in chapter 6.

I will not consider the fatigue resulting from major illnesses in these pages. The exhaustion of the terminal cancers, advanced heart disease and strokes, Parkinsonism, multiple sclerosis, motor neurone disease and many other conditions that present an unambiguous diagnosis should not be included under the CFS umbrella. With many serious diseases, the cause of fatigue and other symptoms is explicit and diagnosable, being clearly obvious to the general practitioner or hospital consultant.

Mitochondrial failure

All human cells consume and produce energy. This universal currency is known as 'adenosine triphosphate' (ATP).

Each cell in the human body contains up to 3000 power units, which are known as the 'mitochondria'. In addition to processing up to 80% of raw materials (our food) into ATP, the mitochondria also distribute our energy. Not surprisingly, many practitioners and researchers consider that mitochondrial function is central to CFS causation, with energy deprivation resulting from mitochondrial failure or malfunction. There is growing interest in the role of mitochondrial malfunction and ATP deficiency in CFS, fibromyalgia and a large range of fatigue-related syndromes.

Dr Paul St Amand (see Further reading, page 251) has claimed that 'widespread metabolic mayhem can all be explained by inadequate sources of ATP'. He also states, 'Only restoration of normal ATP production can give back to patients their mental and physical energies.'

The causes of mitochondrial malfunction are inherited through the female line, but the many mitochondrial inhibitors include stress, poor diets and various toxins, including toxic metals (such as mercury – see pages 81–86) and toxic drugs (such as statins and metformin). Faulty lipid (fat) metabolism can also contribute to mitochondrial deficiency.

Cellular fuel protection and ATP restoration are described in detail in chapter 6, under treatment.

Iron-deficient anaemia (IDA)

A good medical dictionary describes over 90 different anaemias, usually defined according to their cause, but by far the commonest is 'iron-deficient anaemia' (IDA).

In 1986 it was estimated that up to 15% of the world's population had IDA (that is, 500-600 million people). In a recent survey in two teaching hospitals in the UK, up to 50% of IDA was considered to have been either misdiagnosed as other health problems, or gone undiagnosed. Meanwhile, it is thought that in the general population around 10-25% of pre-menopausal women, 1% of men and up to 10% of the elderly of both sexes have IDA.

Unfortunately there is a mistaken belief often encountered in alternative or complementary medicine that GPs are quite able to diagnose and treat IDA. They argue that the tests are simple and unambiguous and the treatment is cheap and effective, the usual prescription being ferrous sulphate, though other iron salts, including ferrous fumarate and gluconate, are also prescribed. With severe iron deficiency, iron injections, iron infusions or even blood transfusions may be prescribed.

Regrettably, I have found in practice that the medical diagnosis and subsequent treatment of IDA are very often flawed and open to question. I have frequently found that fatigued patients actually do have IDA though they have been repeatedly reassured by their GPs – often over several years – that their blood test results are normal and do not indicate iron-deficient anaemia.

How can this happen? Why do so many exhausted patients slip through the long-established medical procedure for diagnosing IDA? I will review this and offer some explanations in chapter 5, on diagnosis (see page 115).

However, it is unlikely that simple iron deficiency would cause the debilitating fatigue typical of CFS, and even less likely for it to cause the galaxy of CFS symptoms. Nevertheless, IDA is often one of the contributing causes of chronic fatigue and it can lead to other symptoms. These include pallor, irritability, poor concentration, headaches, tinnitus (ringing in the ears), indigestion, dyspnoea (shortness of breath), dizziness, leg cramps and heart palpitations. Periods may stop and there may be chest pain and even heart failure. Iron deficiency has also been known to cause pica (a craving for substances other than food, examples being ice and dirt) and can contribute to learning difficulties in children.

Causes of IDA

The chief cause of IDA is blood loss. A standard question for pre-menopausal female patients is therefore, 'Do you have any trouble with your periods?' Excessively heavy (for example, with clotting) or prolonged periods can cause a woman to lose up to 30 milligrams of iron, which is equal to the total iron content of food eaten over four weeks. In men, blood loss usually results from stomach ulceration, intestinal bleeds (such as in Crohn's disease), haemorrhoids or over-enthusiastic use of non-steroid anti-inflammatory drugs (NSAIDS), examples being ibuprofen and aspirin.

Iron is found at high levels in many foods, including red meat (especially liver), shell fish, beans and pulses, some nuts and seeds, and dark green leaf vegetables. Iron deficiency, resulting essentially from an inadequate diet, is relatively rare in western nations. However, certain sections of the population are at risk, this being as a result partly of diet and partly of a greater need for iron, or poor absorption of the mineral. These groups include:

- Infants under two years of age, whose diets are often high in cereals and milk and low in iron-containing foods
- Adolescents who consume insufficient iron as a result of following junk food diets
- Teenage girls after puberty who have excessively heavy periods ('menorrhagia')
- Pregnant women – they have an increased iron requirement, which is not always supplied by their diet
- The elderly – they are at particular risk as a result of decreased ability to absorb iron, and chronic diarrhoea (common in older age)
- Low-income groups as animal protein may be too costly to feature sufficiently in their diet
- In certain vulnerable groups (generally, young enthusiasts) badly designed vegetarian and vegan diets can lead to insufficient iron intake.

It is important to be aware that cow's milk is almost completely deficient in iron. This used to be an issue for infant formula milks, but these are now fortified with iron, and infant IDA is rare in the West. Parents' ongoing worries about iron deficiency and reliance on supplements recently led a reviewer to comment, 'Today's parents are so paranoid about iron deficiency that it is surprising that the typical child can get through an airport without setting off any alarms.'

Understanding iron absorption

For iron to be absorbed from our food the following process needs to take place, with each stage occurring satisfactorily. First, foods are subjected to very high levels of acid in our stomachs; this breaks them down sufficiently for the iron within to become available. (A low gastric acid level, 'hypochlorhydria', can compromise this stage in the process.) Iron is then actually absorbed in the parts of the small intestine called the 'upper jejunum' and 'duodenum'.

Vitamin C is essential for this process to be optimal as it reduces the complex from of iron that is chiefly found in foods to a form that can more easily be absorbed. With age, the lining of the small intestine may atrophy and thereby make iron absorption less efficient.

This process allows only approximately 10% of the iron from our food (around 1 milligram per day) to be absorbed. In healthy adult men and post-menopausal women, normal iron loss is 1 milligram daily via urine, sweat and defecation. Women who are pre-menopausal can lose up to 30 milligrams during their period every month in addition to the 1 mg on ordinary days.

Aside from excessively heavy periods and other causes of blood loss that I have already listed, iron requirements also tend to rise for blood donors and those with a severe stress-load. This can amount to 5 mg per day. Additional requirements for iron during pregnancy can total 7 milligrams per day.

Other dietary influences that are known to reduce availability and absorption of iron include:

- High tea, coffee and chocolate consumption as these all inhibit iron absorption
- Vitamin B-12 and/or folic acid (vitamin B-9) deficiency (see below)
- Vitamin C deficiency as this vitamin plays an essential part in iron absorption
- Deficiency or imbalance in the gut bacteria (leading to inefficient gut permeability)
- Excessive alcohol consumption as alcohol inhibits iron absorption
- Eating calcium-rich foods (such as dairy products) as calcium can reduce iron absorption; it has been shown that women in particular are able to absorb up to 50% more iron from a meal when the calcium content of the meal is low.

Vitamin B-12 deficiency

Vitamin B-12 deficiency causes a whole range of symptoms, of which debilitating fatigue is a key one experienced by most sufferers. It can also lead to breathing difficulties, memory and concentration issues and balance problems. I will describe these in detail below.

Our bodies require 13 different minerals to remain healthy. They are required in very small amounts and are therefore known as 'trace elements'. Vitamin B-12 is unique among the vitamins in that it includes within its chemical structure one of these trace elements – the mineral cobalt. This gives it its scientific name 'cobalamin'. Animals that can produce their own B-12 can do so only if there is enough cobalt in their diets; in Australia, where the soil is deficient in cobalt, farmers provide cobalt 'licks' for their animals as deficiency can cause 'staggers' in cows, similar to the balance problems seen in humans deficient in B-12.

Vitamin B-12 is produced in the gut of animals and is not contained in plants, nor can we synthesise it from sunlight. For us humans to obtain vitamin B-12 from food, we need to eat meat, fish, poultry, eggs or dairy products, or foods that have been 'fortified' by adding vitamin B-12. Although it is well established that those who follow vegan or vegetarian diets and are careless with supplements can become vitamin B-12 deficient, what is less recognised is that many people who do eat foods rich in vitamin B-12 may still deficient in this vitamin. The reason for this paradox lies in the complexity of vitamin B-12 absorption. A problem at any stage in this process can lead to vitamin B-12 deficiency. The digestive pathway can be summarised as follows:

1. When food containing vitamin B-12 arrives in the stomach it is broken down by hydrochloric acid to allow the vitamin to become available for absorption.
2. As vitamin B-12 is what is called a 'protein-bound' substance, an enzyme called 'pepsin' is also needed to extract it from our food.
3. For absorption in the small intestine, another substance needs to be available. This is known as 'intrinsic factor' and is produced by special cells in the stomach lining in healthy people.
4. Proteins known as 'R-binders' are needed to carry the B-12 into the small intestine.
5. In the small intestine, intrinsic factor attaches to the B-12 assisted by additional enzymes – the 'pancreatic proteases'.
6. The B-12 is absorbed into the blood by receptor cells in the part of the small intestine called the 'ileum'.

7.   Finally, 'transcobalamin II', another protein, transports the vitamin B-12 throughout the body.

To understand this process, and the problems that can arise with it, more fully I would recommend two recently published books: *Could it be B12? – an epidemic of misdiagnosis* (by Pacholok & Stuart)and *Pernicious Anaemia – the forgotten disease* (by M Hooper). These are detailed in the Further reading section (see pages 249 and 250).

If we eat more vitamin B-12 than we need, our liver can store sufficient for three to four years. This means that strict vegan diets – which will contain no B-12 – can appear to be 'working' for this length of time before fatigue and other symptoms develop.

Pernicious anaemia and other causes of B-12 deficiency

'Pernicious anaemia', meaning anaemia that kills, is just one cause of B-12 deficiency. It should be suspected in people who eat plenty of B-12 but still suffer from the symptoms of the deficiency. It is an auto-immune condition that is often inherited and results in the decreased production of intrinsic factor, which we know from the process described above is essential for B-12 absorption and, ultimately, the production of red blood cells.

There are, however, many more common causes of vitamin B-12 deficiency. These include various types of gastritis (inflammation of the stomach lining), which can reduce available stomach acid, infections or surgery. Certain drugs can also cause 'erosive gastritis' – for example, the NSAIDs (non-steroid anti-inflammatories), such as ibuprofen and aspirin.

Atrophic gastritis is common in the elderly. It involves inflammation and deterioration of the stomach lining and a subsequent reduction in stomach acid. Stomach surgery can cause a reduction in both the cells that produce the stomach acid, hydrochloric acid, and those that produce intrinsic factor. Other causes include Crohn's disease (intestinal inflammation), coeliac disease (gluten intolerance), excessive intake of alcohol (as with iron-deficient anaemia), mercury toxicity and exposure to nitrous oxide ('laughing gas') either during surgery or dentistry, or in recreational use.

With vitamin B-12 deficiency, the important fact to remember is that many people who are deficient in B-12 do in fact consume plenty of B-12 in their food. Their real problem is that, for a variety of reasons, they cannot absorb vitamin B-12 in sufficient amounts.

Symptoms of vitamin B-12 deficiency

Vitamin B-12 deficiency has been termed 'the great imitator'. There is no such thing as a typical B-12 syndrome. Deficiency can produce symptoms in all the body systems. Below I will summarise the signs and symptoms, but they are not unique to B-12 deficiency; other possible causes should always be considered.

All these symptoms tend to be slow to develop. This, as Martyn Hooper explains in *Pernicious Anaemia – the forgotten disease*, can lead sufferers to blame their symptoms on life-style pressures, their age, their family history and other factors, without any awareness of actual ill-health. It does not help that the descriptions of these symptoms in medical textbooks tend to be imprecise.

- **Fatigue** – Fatigue is, of course, our primary focus in this book. The tiredness experienced by those deficient in vitamin B-12 has been defined as 'the strange tiredness', a fatigue that is not relieved by sleep. In fact, waking up tired is a common complaint.
- **Breathing difficulties** – Aside from fatigue, another common symptom group includes breathing difficulties, often indicated by frequent sighing and yawning.
- **Memory and concentration** – poor short-term memory and confusion with marked absent-mindedness are also typical symptoms.
- **Balance problems** – poor balance, pins and needles (paraesthesia), usually in the legs and feet, and numbness in the legs can occur. Vertigo and very poor balance when standing with eyes closed.

Unfortunately such symptoms do not always improve or clear when the blood vitamin B-12 level is raised to an acceptable level by means of injections of B-12. This, in my opinion, tends to highlight the overlap of many symptoms with CFS. The symptoms linked to low vitamin B-12 are very similar to the 'hypo' symptoms caused by adrenal fatigue with subsequent low blood sugar (see chapter 6, adrenal fatigue (page 193) and low blood sugar (see page 215)). This may explain why normalising a patient's blood B-12 level does not always eliminate the symptoms as described – there are other underlying problems that also need to be addressed.

Vitamin B-12 deficiency has the potential to compromise the function of many organs and systems. The symptoms as outlined above are not specific to B-12 deficiency, but can be caused by other disorders. However, it does make sense to consider vitamin B-12 deficiency as one possible cause that can contribute to CFS symptoms and to rule out or treat this common problem.

Organs and body systems influenced by B-12 deficiency

- **Blood** – the body cannot make sufficient healthy red blood cells to carry appropriate levels of oxygen around the body, resulting in anaemia, fatigue, shortness of breath (dyspnoea), enlarged liver and/or spleen, enlarged red blood cells.
- **Immune system** – increased liability to infections and poor response to vaccines; poor wound healing.
- **Bowel** – abdominal discomfort and pain, indigestion and fullness, gastric reflux, constipation and/or diarrhoea.
- **Genital and reproductive systems** – bladder incontinence, impotence, infertility.
- **Muscles and skeleton** – osteoporosis and a tendency for bones to fracture easily.
- **Nervous system** – numbness, paraesthesia (pins and needles) of extremities, general clumsiness with falling, poor balance. Burning sensation in limbs, tremor, mental confusion, depression and absent-mindedness, headaches and hallucinations, violent behaviour.
- **Vascular** – blood clots (pulmonary embolism), deep vein thrombosis (DVT) of the extremities, strokes and transient ischaemic attacks or mini-strokes (TIAs).
- Palpitations, hypotension (low blood pressure) when standing.

You will appreciate that vitamin B-12 can cause malfunctioning of almost all the body organs and systems.

Underactive thyroid (hypothyroidism)

An under-functioning thyroid gland is one of the most common causes of chronic fatigue. One of my earlier books (*Why Am I So Tired?*) focuses on hypothyroidism; as a consequence, I probably see more thyroid patients than the average naturopath, as many people have consulted me after reading the book.

The thyroid gland, situated in the throat, is a component of the 'endocrine axis'. This comprises the hypothalamus (within the brain), the pituitary gland, the thyroid, the adrenal glands and the ovaries or testes; this chain of glands is under the overall control of the hypothalamus.

The thyroid gland controls our metabolic rate, and every organ in the body can suffer if the thyroid is underactive. The human thyroid can vary in weight from 8 to 50 grams. There are also wide variations in thyroid function among 'normal' human beings. Such variables help to account for why a diagnosis of hypothyroidism is often missed as a possible factor in chronic fatigue.

The medical diagnosis of underactive thyroid is based almost entirely on blood test results, which are themselves judged according to 'normal' range assessments. This in particular involves the levels of the hormones known as 'free T4' (thyroxine) and 'TSH' (thyroid stimulating hormone, produced by the pituitary gland) in the blood. In European laboratories, and especially those used by the UK's National Health Service, the normal ranges for free T4 are amongst the lowest in the world. This ensures that many patients with CFS with borderline or low thyroid output are not thought to need treatment. The chief diagnostic test requested for hypothyroidism is usually the TSH test (TSH levels rise to stimulate an inefficient thyroid), but I regard this as unfortunate because TSH will often only increase with well-established, severe hypothyroidism, allowing borderline conditions again to be missed.

All these factors contribute to GPs discounting the possibility that underactive thyroid could be partly or entirely to blame for their patients' chronic fatigue.

I shall return to this 'black or white' diagnostic protocol elsewhere in the book. The two important concepts of biochemical individuality and possible functional inefficiency are discounted or ignored in favour of looking for a specific disease or damage. A patient's symptoms are not seen as a contributing, worthwhile factor in making a diagnosis.

I have seen very exhausted patients who have been taking thyroxine for many years and and have been frequently reassured that they are not hypothyroid. Their test results usually turn out to fall within the normal range, yet with treatment and a subsequent increase in their blood level of free T4, their symptoms often improve.

What about T3?

Many of my fatigued thyroid patients have asked me, 'What about T3?' Very often these patients have been prescribed and been taking T4 (thyroxine) for several years without much improvement in their symptoms. They have learned, probably from books or the internet, that it is the hormone T3, known as 'triiodothyronine', that is the most biologically active thyroid hormone, yet it is very rarely prescribed. Up to 80% of the T3 in our blood results from the conversion of T4 to T3, chiefly in the liver and kidneys. Only around 20% of the T3 we use is actually produced by the thyroid gland. For this reason, there are many hypothyroid patients who achieve benefit solely from a prescription of T4 – but they must be able to convert T4 to T3.

Conversion of T4 to T3 depends on enzymes called 'deiodinases' *within our cells*. (It is very important to note that thyroid hormones have to be in our cells to work; those circulating in the blood do not contribute to our energy needs.) Without the thyroid hormone entering our cells and an adequate supply of deodinases, we cannot make use of T4. Many practitioners who regularly treat hypothyroid patients believe that providing a combination of T4 and T3 can be more effective than T4 alone, whether blood levels appear to be normal or not.

This combination treatment can be effective for chronic fatigue, fibromyalgia and depression. For many CFS patients who are taking T4, their continuing fatigue points to poor conversion of T4 to T3, resulting in the failure of their T4 pill to provide adequate and normal brain and body functioning. This is one explanation for the common scenario of 'normal' test results, but persisting symptoms. Supplements are available to assist the conversion of T4 to T3, such as T-Convert produced by Nutri-Advanced.

In spite of the proven benefit of the 'combination' approach to hypothyroidism, a recent book, *Recovering with T3* by Paul Robinson, includes the following comment: 'T3 replacement therapy should only be used after all other forms of thyroid hormone replacement have been exhausted.' He further states that, 'I am hoping that the medical profession will begin to consider the use of the T3 as a more mainstream and valuable thyroid medication than it appears to do at the present time.' Treatment must be approached in a systematic way, trying one option, then another – I have seen patients who have self-prescribed and purchased T3 and T4 on the internet and had many problems with their thyroid symptoms in consequence. Such views tend to confirm the individual complexity of diagnosing and treating the underactive thyroid. Fortunately, the thyroid glandulars (see Glossary, page 262) can provide the precursor nutrients (again, see Glossary) for all the thyroid hormones. I find that these can often succeed in providing symptom relief for patients who are taking T4 but not experiencing symptom improvement.

Wilson's syndrome

Dr E Denis Wilson, an American physician, chose to name a form of thyroid illness after himself. He controversially suggested that the conversion of T4 to T3 was at times inefficient, leading to a patient suffering symptoms but with normal test results (this being termed 'sick euthyroid syndrome', with 'euthyroid' meaning 'normal thyroid'.) The existence of this syndrome is not recognised by conventional medicine.

Reverse T3

'Reverse T3' was only recognised in the 1950s. Its chief function is to control any surplus T3. Its power and effect on our metabolism are minimal, T4 being around 20 times more effective. It can decrease our ability to convert T4 to T3 in the event of starvation, serious illness and high levels of stress. However, as a hormone it is not independently biologically active.

Lupus erythematosus

Systemic lupus erythematosus (SLE) is the commonest of over 15 types of lupus. Lupus is a chronic auto-immune disorder with periods of remission, often misdiagnosed as rheumatoid arthritis, multiple sclerosis or CFS. Blood tests can assist diagnosis. The connective tissue (tendons etc) is chiefly affected. Symptoms can include fatigue, anaemia, joint and muscle pain, sensitivity to sunlight, and kidney, skin, spleen and heart disorders.

SLE can be drug induced, and silicone breast implants have been known to be a cause. For many types of lupus, however, the cause is unknown.

Treatment can include anti-inflammatory drugs, anticoagulants and corticosteroids.

Adrenal fatigue ('hypoadrenalism' or 'hypoadrenia')

Adrenal fatigue, sometimes called 'non-Addison's hypoadrenia', is an increasingly common condition. It plays a major part in causing fatigue as it results in the under functioning of the adrenal system. I will describe below how this comes about. It should not to be confused with 'Addison's disease', which is a rare condition involving auto-immune destruction of the outer-layer of the adrenal gland that leads to deficiency in the vital adrenal hormones, chiefly cortisol. Addison's disease can be fatal in the absence of prescribed hormone replacement therapy.

The adrenal system consists of two small glands varying in weight from 7 to 20 grams, located adjacent to the top of each kidney. The outer layer of the glands, known as the 'cortex', secretes many steroid hormones, including cortisone, cortisol, DHEA (dehydroepiandrosterone), pregnenolone, aldosterone and the androgens. The androgens serve as precursor hormones (see Glossary) to the sex hormones, testosterone and the oestrogens. The inner part of the adrenals, known as the 'medulla', secretes adrenaline (epinephrine) and nor-adrenaline (nor-epinephrine). To understand the complex actions of these hormones and why their deficiency leads to chronic fatigue I have summarised them in the box on page 53.

The methods for testing a patient's adrenal status are the subject of some controversy. The test for Addison's disease, which is virtually the only test routinely requested by the medical establishment, is the 'synacthen test'. However, while this test is extremely sensitive to primary adrenal insufficiency, it is significantly less so to secondary adrenal insufficiency; consequently, many people with secondary insufficiency are erroneously given a 'normal' result. If a patient does not test positive then he or she will be discharged as being 'healthy'. Fortunately, alternative medicine recognises tests for another form of hypoadrenia – that caused by adrenal deficiency

THE ROLE OF THE ADRENAL HORMONES

Hormones are produced by the medulla and the cortex

MEDULLA – Central 1

Hormones
Adrenalin (Epinephrine)
Noradrenalin (Norepinephrine)

Functions
Rapid stress response
(sometimes referred to as 'fight or flight')

CORTEX – 2-3-4
Zona reticularis – inner layer 2

Hormones
DHEA
Pregnenolone
Progesterones,Oestrogens,
Testosterones (Androgens)

Functions
Sex hormone precursor
DHEA and sex hormone precursor

Sex hormones
Can indicate biological age

Zona fasciculata – middle layer 3

Hormone
Cortisol
(Therapeutically – hydrocortisone)

Functions
Regulates blood sugar
Anti-inflammatory
Immune response support
Aids stress reaction
Affects protein and fat metabolism

Zona glomerulosa – outer layer 4

Hormone
Aldosterone

Functions
Assists regulation of sodium, potassium
and body fluids

The adrenal layers

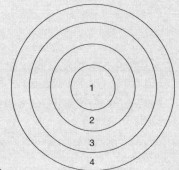

1. Medulla
2. ⎫ Zona reticularis
3. ⎬ Cortex Zona fasciculata
4. ⎭ Zona glomerulosa

or fatigue. This is diagnosed using the 'adrenal stress profile' test, which provides information on levels of cortisol and DHEA. This involves testing four samples of a person's saliva taken over a 15-16 hour period in a single day, and can be done at home. I routinely request my CFS patients to have this test. Although only two of the many adrenal hormones are measured, by doing so the test provides a general view of adrenal efficiency.

With the complexity and great variety of adrenal hormones, you will not be surprised that reduced adrenal function or fatigue can contribute to a huge variety of symptoms.

Common symptoms of adrenal fatigue (not in order of frequency or severity)

Low blood pressure with dizziness upon standing
Headaches
Low blood sugar (hypoglycaemia)
Fatigue
Feeling stressed
Craving for salt and sugar-rich foods
Poor memory and concentration
Fatigue worse on rising
Poor alcohol and caffeine tolerance
Insomnia
Poor exercise tolerance with muscle weakness
Frequent infections
Dark patches under the eyes
Generally shaky and weak
Poor stress-handling and panic attacks
Fluid retention but sweaty hands when nervous
PMS (pre-menstrual syndrome) symptoms (irritability, fatigue, sugar-
     craving and fluid retention) tend to worsen
Reduced libido (sex drive)
Generally worse with delayed or missed meals
Depression and anxiety.

Chapter 3

Adrenal fatigue – the causes

The chief cause of adrenal fatigue is stress (for example, see *Adrenal Fatigue* by James Wilson). Such stress is not just from the obvious causes, such as a dispute with a neighbour, employment problems or family arguments. There are many different forms of stress. Quite simply, the adrenals can become exhausted when our stress load exceeds the capacity of these glands to compensate for and recover from the stress. Stress can be emotional, psychological, environmental, physical or infectious. However, our stress usually consists of a mixture of different stress sources. Unfortunately many of those who suffer from chronic fatigue, perhaps over several years, can be trapped in a vicious circle of exhaustion, anxiety and pain, leading to further additional stress. The symptoms themselves can become part of their stress load. We need to realise that our adrenal system responds in a similar way to *every* kind of stress whatever the origin of the stress may be.

There is a tendency to look on the stress in our lives as essentially anything that can cause unhappiness, anxiety or fatigue, yet it is important to be aware that poor diet, allergies, insufficient – or excessive – exercise, overworking, environmental toxins, excessive caffeine, alcohol and tobacco use, chronic infections and insomnia are all included in a long list of stress causation. The 'dripping tap' variety of stress can be more destructive than a sudden shock.

We all have our own personal ability and potential to manage our stress-load. Time and circumstances can cause this capacity to reduce. The case history (Barbara's story) in chapter 6 (see page 196) serves to demonstrate the value of the adrenal stress profile test, when requested to diagnose and assist treatment requirements. The results, when interpreted, can confirm for the patient that their stress is not 'all in the mind' or a personality defect. When their low adrenal status is confirmed, it can be very reassuring to 'match' the symptoms with the test results, also in a similar way to monitor progress and eventually break the vicious circle discussed earlier. It is of value to identify a treatable problem. In addition, when symptom relief has been achieved, a final test that confirms normal adrenal capacity can be very encouraging to a recovering patient.

When the adrenal reserves (the potential to deal with stress) become depleted as a result of long-term stress, often with several causes, any treatment needs to be on various levels to normalise adrenal efficiency. This is explained further in chapter 6 on Treatment.

Fatigue and the mind (the effects of stress)

Mind-body or psychosomatic disorders have been recognised for over 80 years in medical thinking. The seminal book, *The Stress of Life* by Hans Selye, is often quoted as the main work that defines the concept of stress and presents a unified theory, explaining just how stress can affect our physical health. The adrenal glands are the main system for handling stress. They are also involved in blood sugar control. Not surprisingly, stressed people tend to be fatigued – more later.

Dysthymia (depressive neurosis)

'Dysthymia' describes a very common, but mild form of depression. It is characterised by low mood, fatigue and insomnia. Sufferers are notably unsociable and irritable. It has been defined as creating the 'glass half empty' type of personality. Such pessimism can run through a family and it is often accompanied by anxiety.

Those with dysthymia can go undiagnosed and untreated for decades. Symptoms often begin in the teens. The cause is thought to be a lack of serotonin, a brain neurotransmitter. Although serotonin levels can be measured in the blood, this does not reflect the amount needed for effective brain metabolism.

The medical treatment for dysthymia is usually anti-depressant drugs and cognitive behavioural therapy (CBT). However, a recent study suggests that only one in seven patients actually benefits from anti-depressants. 'Clinical depression' is the term currently in use to define just two weeks of low mood. Mental illness has been aptly defined as 'the drug industry's golden goose'. Fortunately there are alternatives; as with all the forms of depression, the nutrient 5-hydroxytryptophan (5-HTP), which is the natural precursor of serotonin, can be very effective.

Schmidt's syndrome

Schmidt's syndrome, or 'polyglandular autoimmune syndrome type II' (PGA-II), is a condition characterised by combined adrenal and thyroid insufficiency. The chief symptoms are muscle cramping and pain, with fatigue. Tests usually show low cortisol levels and borderline hypothyroidism. The adrenal hormone aldosterone can also be depleted, with increased blood potassium as a result. In young patients, Addison's disease is sometimes suspected.

Fibromyalgia syndrome (FMS)

'Fibromyalgia syndrome' is yet another illness that can cause chronic fatigue and is seen as a member of the CFS, ME and PVF family of conditions. It has been described as 'exhaustion with pain'. Originally termed 'fibrositis' or rheumatism, it represents a syndrome that includes debilitating fatigue and widespread pain. It has also been called an 'invisible disability' as there are no specific diagnostic tests, X-rays or scans to identify the condition or even confirm its existence.

In 1993, the World Health Organisation (WHO) officially declared fibromyalgia to be a 'syndrome'. The condition was thus validated and defined as probably the most frequently seen cause of widespread chronic muscle pain. After this official definition, fibromyalgia became an illness that could be considered by medical insurance. The WHO also added to the definition the following statement: 'Fibromyalgia is part of a wider syndrome encompassing headaches, irritable bladder, dysmenorrhoea (period pain), cold sensitivity, Raynaud's phenomenon, restless legs, a typical numbness and tingling patterns, exercise intolerance, general weakness and depression.'

Fibromyalgia as a diagnosis continues to be disputed in medicine as there is rarely any muscle or joint damage to detect, and scans and X-rays show negative results. However, specific tender points on the body have been identified. These are known as 'trigger points'. Eighteen points have been defined as typical and finding the points has been termed as 'mapping'.

Unfortunately, a diagnosis of fibromyalgia can take up to 18 months to confirm from the onset of symptoms to the eventual diagnosis. Officially it remains 'incurable' and many doctors still see it as a neurotic menopausal-woman's complaint, though there is evidence that it is the most frequent condition seen by rheumatologists. It mainly affects the elderly and is 10 times more common in women than in men. In a recent book (*What Your Doctor May Not Tell You About Fibromyalgia*), one of the authors (R Paul St

Amand, an American endocrinologist who has specialised in the treatment of fibromyalgia over a 50 year career) states that up to 5% of the adult American population can be seen as fibromyalgia sufferers. This amounts to 26 million people. (Another author, Dr Chris Jenner, estimated the number more conservatively at 12.9 million in 2011.)

So what are the causes of this baffling complaint that seems to combine CFS with muscular rheumatism and a host of other symptoms?

Fibromyalgia – the causes

Pain and fatigue are typical symptoms of thyroid and adrenal hormone deficiencies. Even borderline hypothyroidism and adrenal fatigue with low cortisol can contribute to the symptoms of fibromyalgia. The gender bias of 10 female patients to one male is common to thyroid and adrenal symptoms as well as to fibromyalgia. I have found that approximately 60% of my patients who have a diagnosed thyroid deficiency also experience FM-type symptoms.

The phosphate factor

A single definitive laboratory test profile has yet to be designed to diagnose fibromyalgia. The diversity of symptoms and the variation in their severity from patient to patient have been defined as 'metabolic mayhem' by Paul St Amand. He has pioneered a treatment approach for fibromyalgia patients that is based on removing excess amounts of inorganic phosphate from the cells. These inorganic phosphates may build up at this level as the result of an inherited kidney malfunction or defective cellular enzymes. Excess phosphates can reduce mitochondrial function so their removal may release energy that has been previously blocked. Having treated thousands of patients and achieved symptom-relief in around 90%, he and his colleagues offer convincing evidence to confirm their methodology.

So what exactly is the connection between phosphate, body energy and fibromyalgia symptoms? The link may be adenosine triphosphate (ATP), the universal energy currency produced by the mitrochondria within our cells (see earlier in this chapter, page 40). Many researchers and physicians believe that only by normalising ATP production can our mental and physical energy normalise. CFS is often seen as a symptom of mitochondrial failure. I have described the available tests for measuring ATP status and cellular energy in chapter 5, on diagnosis (see page 119).

Excess phosphate is thought to block or reduce ATP production in the mitochondria, thus causing the symptoms of fibromyalgia. Unfortunately, the reduced ATP present in patients with fibromyalgia syndrome also allows calcium to build up. This in turn leads to localised swelling and the characteristic 'trigger pain points' of the condition.

As with so many variants of CFS that I have seen, causes are complex: fibromyalgia syndrome is not simply a result of phosphate blockage. Sufferers usually also have adrenal imbalance with low blood sugar to contribute to the muscle/joint pain and their chronic fatigue.

Candidiasis (the 'yeast syndrome')

'Candidiasis' is the term used for yeast overgrowth in the gut. Yeasts are single-cell fungi that normally and harmlessly live in the tissue lining the human gut, from mouth to rectum, the gut 'mucous membrane'. There are over 100 species of candidia, by far the commonest being *Candida albicans*. When these yeasts 'over grow' in the vagina, rectum or throat, many practitioners see this problem as an irritating but superficial condition, commonly known as 'thrush'. However, 'systemic candidiasis' is a rather more serious problem. This describes an increase in the yeast, often as a result of excessive antibiotic use, birth-control pills or steroid drugs. When this occurs, the yeasts threaten a person's immune system with the release of toxins. This can influence virtually all the body's organs, even the brain. Although CFS is unlikely to be caused solely by candidiasis, the list of symptoms serves to illustrate the similarity between systemic candidiasis and many CFS symptoms.

Candidiasis symptoms:

Hormonal symptoms
Thyroid, oestrogen/progesterone and adrenal disturbance
Mental/emotional symptoms
Mood changes, poor short-term memory, anxiety, depression, 'foggy'
headaches and irritability

Immunity problems
Chemical sensitivities and allergies, histamine excess and generally
poor immune response to infections
Digestive symptoms
Stomach fullness (gas), thrush, irritable bowel syndrome (IBS), rectal
itch, diarrhoea and constipation, heartburn, sore throat, mouth and
tongue, colic and haemorrhoids
General symptoms
Fatigue, reduced libido, skin disorders, fluid retention, cystitis, joint and
muscle pains, fungal 'infections' of the nails, headaches and low
blood sugar.

The general view of candidiasis is that it is a 'woman's complaint' that
can cause vaginal thrush and cystitis. It can generally be cured with a course
of the anti-fungal drug nystatin and any symptoms are usually local and
short term. Unfortunately, for many vulnerable sufferers it can be a major
contributing cause of the range of symptoms listed, particularly fatigue and
immune system breakdown. HIV positive patients have been known to
develop candidiasis of the brain.

As with so many facets of the CFS story, candidiasis requires specific
testing to identify its severity, coupled with a thorough supplement and
nutritional programme in order to eliminate this very stubborn and frequently
chronic condition. Treatment is described in chapter 6 (see page 207).

Problems with digestion

Whenever I see new patients for their initial consultation, I always try to find
time to discuss their eating and drinking habits. In spite of the adverse views
of many celebrity cooks, chefs and food writers, I believe that the British diet
has improved over the last 50 years. This particularly applies to food quality
and diversity. The major food retailers frequently use words like 'green',
'natural', 'organic' and 'free-range' to support their offerings, obviously with
the knowledge that quality sells, provided people have the budget. Yet, I am
frequently asked by exhausted patients why they feel so tired when they eat

wholesome food. I usually respond by pointing out that filling a faulty car with high octane fuel does not guarantee happy motoring.

So, in spite of the food and cookery sections in many national newspapers and well over a dozen cookery magazines being available, why are digestive problems so widespread? I should not forget the cookery quizzes, demonstrations and food-based travel programmes that are scheduled on TV nightly.

I believe there are several clear reasons for the frequency of irritable bowel syndrome (IBS), bowel disease, hypochlorhydria, gastritis, constipation, reflux, diarrhoea and nausea, the modern high-sugar diet being chief among them. Furthermore, such disorders and symptoms are often central to the development of CFS; our conversion of food to energy can be compromised by them; it is therefore appropriate to include them as a contributing cause of CFS.

The link between energy and digestion

Many of us see energy use expressed as muscle movement and activity, examples being walking, running and talking. However, all the functions of our metabolism need energy, in particular breathing, digesting food, brain use and immune support. Approximately 85% of our food needs to be converted to energy and we need an efficient digestive system do this.

What is clear is that to ensure an optimum energy supply we need quality food, efficient digestion and absorption, and regular and reliable elimination. Our gut environment in terms of enzyme status, the acid-alkali balance and the presence of friendly intestinal bacteria needs to be protected and effective. (Our total beneficial gut bacteria colony weighs around six pounds.) The question remains, why can those on a balanced, nutrient-rich diet develop CFS? As you will by now be aware, there are many conditions that can contribute to chronic fatigue. Digestive disorders are usually only part of the jigsaw puzzle. A catalogue of commonly found digestive conditions in CFS is as follows.

'Hypochlorhydria' (hydrochloric acid (HCl) deficiency)

Hydrochloric acid in the stomach is essential for efficient protein digestion and to sterilise the food we have eaten by killing random microbes. It has been estimated that around 10–20% of people over 60 years do not produce enough hydrochloric acid, although younger people can also have this problem. The symptoms resulting from low acid status include stomach fullness with flatulence (belching), and nausea when taking supplements. Food transit (the passage of food from mouth to rectum) is delayed and the whole digestive system is slowed down. Undigested food can often be seen in the stools. Although low stomach acid is not the only cause of indigestion, it has been known to exacerbate food allergies, diabetes, iron and vitamin B-12 deficient anaemias, candidiasis, bowel infections and various skin and joint problems.

Efficient protein digestion is an important requirement for the absorption of vitamins and minerals and many other nutrients, an example being the B vitamin, folic acid, which we cannot absorb unless our protein digestion is effective. The supplement *Betain HCl with pepsin* can normally increase stomach acidity to support digestion. However, I advise readers to consult a practitioner about this.

Reduced pancreatic enzymes

An important role of the pancreas, and other organs in the body, is to produce enzymes – complex chemical compounds that enable metabolic processes in our bodies to take place. The pancreas produces a number of enzymes that are vital for digestion. When these enzymes are deficient, digestion becomes faulty and symptoms can arise.

In the human digestive system, food (of any type) leaves the stomach and enters the small intestine. This organ is around 20 feet in length and food is absorbed via its walls, after being broken down by the action of the pancreatic enzymes. It may help to supplement these and formulas are often combined with *Betain HCl* and 'ox-bile' (a safe and effective supplement, despite its unpleasant name) to ensure fats, proteins and carbohydrates are effectively broken down. The bile salts in the ox-bile are essential for fat digestion. Fats are a potent energy source and the poor digestion of fats causes symptoms, including foul-smelling stools that float, bowel gas and the inevitable fatigue. The chief symptom linked to enzyme deficiency is, once more, fatigue.

Leaky gut ('intestinal hyperpermeability')

When our digestion is impaired, undigested molecules can cause a condition known as 'leaky gut syndrome'. Although this common condition is unlikely to be a major cause of CFS, it can be one of the many contributing factors. Part of our defence system is the intestinal mucosa or barrier that lines our gut from end to end. When this barrier is compromised, foreign substances, including the candidas and other yeasts and funguses, and incompletely digested foods, particularly proteins, can enter the blood stream. There are many causes that contribute to this syndrome. These include candidiasis, food allergies, nutritional deficiencies, excessive alcohol consumption, excessive sugar in the diet, steroid and anti-inflammatory drugs (NSAIDs), food additives and reduced beneficial gut bacteria resulting from antibiotic use. I describe the diagnosis and treatment of the leaky gut syndrome in detail in chapters 5 (page 129) and 6 (page 209).

Food allergies and intolerances

You may wonder just what is the difference between an allergy and an intolerance. Both terms refer to an area of digestive ill-health that is widespread and yet controversial. It is only in recent years that medical testing, diagnosis and treatment of food allergies have become standardised and effective. The terms used to define food and environmental sensitivities (allergy and intolerance) are virtually interchangeable.

It has been estimated that food allergies alone cause symptoms in around 2% of the adult population and 8% of children. Environmental allergies can result from exposure to pesticides, food additives, drugs and the many toxins that are present in our food. Water pollutants (including chlorine and fluoride) account for many more symptoms in the population.

The exclusion–reintroduction diet
Aside from food breakdown and absorption, our digestive system offers the first line of defence against many allergens. Not surprisingly, if our fuel supply is compromised, fatigue is one of the many symptoms that will occur. Other common symptoms caused by food intolerances include IBS, headaches, sinusitis, skin disorders, fibromyalgia, arthritis and auto-immune conditions.

Such food triggers can often be identified by the use of an exclusion diet. This is a diet that avoids known trigger foods. These typically include grains, chocolate, sugar, peanuts, eggs and dairy products. Assuming there is some symptom-relief after following this exclusion programme for three to four weeks, the next step involves a systematic reintroduction of the foods one at a time, to identify any symptom reccurrence. The object is to link symptoms with specific foods. The full programme is discussed in chapter 6 (see page 213).

Post-viral fatigue (PVF)

Post-viral fatigue (PVF) is recognised as a cause of CFS. Although 'chronic fatigue syndrome' (CFS) is an umbrella term for debilitating, long-term fatigue, in the UK, PVF is also known as 'myalgic encephalomyelitis' (ME), whilst in America the name used is 'chronic fatigue and immune dysfunction syndrome' (CFIDS).The common theme to these names is that they all imply that a problem with immunity contributes to the fatigue.

Current theories pointing to the causes of PVF include a virus (often polio-related) or environmental factors, including toxic contamination of our food, soil, air and water. Although a viral cause of CFS has been researched for around 80 years, recent evidence has failed to confirm this as a cause of PVF (ME). However, I have seen many patients who can trace the onset of their symptoms to a particular infection. This is usually a 'flu-like infection or glandular fever (mononucleosis).

Parasites

I have also talked to those who have experienced unusual fatigue following a holiday in India, Thailand or other eastern countries. This is usually caused by parasites, which can be transmitted in food and drinking water and by insects. Food poisoning resulting in bouts of acute diarrhoea can also cause chronic fatigue. Such causes of long-term fatigue are quite common.

I routinely request details of recent holidays, or of 'gap-years' experienced by students and other young travellers (see Valerie's story in chapter 6, page 221). Young 'back-packers' cannot usually afford to stay in large hotels in city centres, so they are more vulnerable to water- and food-borne infections in the rural areas that they visit.

The investigation of this possible diagnosis, and the subsequent treatment for such a cause of fatigue, calls for meticulous case-history taking. Unfortunately, the evidence from tests can be unsatisfactory or non-existent.

Low blood sugar (hypoglycaemia)

We have all experienced symptoms of low blood sugar, although without always being aware of the cause. Examples of these symptoms include:

- Feeling shaky and tired if a meal has been missed or you have gone without food for 4-5 hours
- Feeling tired and irritable on waking and often feeling more vital at the end of the day
- In women, pre-menstrual symptoms, particularly a craving for chocolate, are often caused by falls in the blood sugar level.

Diabetics who rely on regular insulin injections can misjudge their requirements and overdose on the insulin causing a 'hypo', when blood sugar levels fall dangerously low. The overdose of insulin results in 'hyperinsulinism' (in Greek 'hypo' means below and 'hyper' means above), which in turn results in a slump in the blood sugar (hypoglycaemia). This is usually a transient effect. Diabetic patients learn to avoid 'hypo' situations by carefully balancing their insulin dosages, their diet and their energy output, at the same time regularly checking their blood glucose levels. Diabetic 'hypos' can be very distressing, with severe fatigue, headache, loss of balance, poor concentration, irritability and even collapse and unconsciousness.

In the 1920s, Dr Seale Harris – a general practitioner working in Alabama in the USA – noted that several of his patients exhibited hypo symptoms on a regular basis. However, these people were not diabetic and were therefore not injecting insulin. His reasoning led him to conclude that many glands can be 'hypo' or 'hyper' active, and under-activity (hypo) is often preceded by over-activity (hyper).

Dr Harris was a contemporary of Banting and Best, the co-discoverers of the role of insulin in diabetes. Dr Banting met with Seale Harris and he agreed that his observations represented a new aspect to the study of blood sugar levels.

When I wrote my first book in 1981, *Low Blood Sugar (Hypoglycaemia)*, the subject of non-diabetic sugar 'hypos' was rarely discussed. Since then I have written two further books on low blood sugar and diet, and hypoglycaemia is now recognised as a very common phenomenon and a frequent cause of fatigue. It may result from adrenal fatigue or from a diet high in sugar and carbohydrates. The average diet in Europe and North America is currently sugar-rich, and coffee and alcohol intake are at record highs. Diabetes is increasing as are the low blood sugar symptoms.

In addition to the insulin factor, the adrenal glands are an important component in controlling our blood sugar levels. Insulin lowers the blood sugar but the adrenal hormones raise it. Exhausted, overworked adrenals tend to allow the blood sugar to remain low for long periods, thus adding to the sugar craving. This gives rise to the characteristic fatigue-on-rising symptom that is caused by a fall in blood sugar as a result of the night fast (often 10–12 hours) coupled with an inefficient adrenal response. When our blood sugar falls too low the adrenal response is the same as the 'fight or flight' response to stress. This means that the person feels threatened and the result of this is aggression and irritability. The same sequence of events occurs with many women before a period ('pre-menstrual syndrome' – PMS) and in both sexes when excessive alcohol destabilises the blood sugar.

I always ask my CFS patients, 'How do you feel on rising?' The answer for perhaps 90–95% is, 'Much worse.' They usually only begin to feel normal after breakfast. The best time of day is often early evening. A commonly heard comment about a person, both at home and in the office, is, 'He/she is not worth talking to before breakfast.' However, although the fatigue resulting from this problem can be a major cause of symptoms over many years, it is not a life-threatening condition and as a result does not receive the attention it deserves.

I describe the diagnosis and treatment for low blood sugar in chapters 5 (see page 134) and 6 (see page 215).

Chapter 3

Syndrome X (the metabolic syndrome)

This recently identified syndrome is seen by many doctors and researchers as a major stepping-stone to type II diabetes and many other disorders. It is considered as a risk factor for type II diabetes for around 25% of the populations of the western nations – that is, up to 25% are thought to have the potential to develop syndrome X as they reach middle age.

Syndrome X, or the 'metabolic syndrome', was first defined by Dr Gerald Reaven at the Stanford University School of Medicine in the USA in 2000. It is characterised by insulin resistance (explained below), glucose intolerance (again, explained below), hyperinsulinism (raised blood insulin), high blood fats (triglycerides), low 'good' cholesterol (HDL), high blood pressure and, in women, 'polycystic ovary syndrome' (PCOS). A typical sufferer will be overweight with an enlarged waist measurement and excessive abdominal fat.

Syndrome X is known to be a major contributor to coronary heart disease, strokes, colon and breast cancer, dementia and gout. Unfortunately, with increased abdominal fat around the pancreas and liver, insulin sensitivity tends to decrease and blood sugar control becomes inefficient (glucose intolerance).

Insulin resistance explained

Insulin resistance is a component of syndrome X. It is characterised by a raised level of insulin in the blood (usually caused by a high sugar intake) as a result of the body's cells becoming less sensitive to the action of insulin; as the cells become less sensitive, the body produces more and more insulin to compensate. Unfortunately, one effect of such a rise is increased production of androgens by the female ovaries. This contributes to PCOS, another syndrome with obesity as a major symptom.

Another result of high blood insulin is 'glucose intolerance', the factor behind type ll diabetes, where glucose can no longer be managed by the body. Excessive blood insulin also spurs the liver to produce more triglycerides (blood fat), which are a major risk for heart disease and strokes.

The recent massive increase in syndrome X, obesity and diabetes has been a result of the current western diet, which includes food never previously consumed by humans, in particular, high-fructose corn syrup (HFCS) and trans-fatty acids. The syndrome also interferes with the regulation of many hormones leading to imbalances in thyroid, adrenal and sex hormones and pancreatic secretions.

Infections and acute illness are no longer the chief causes of death in the 21st century, having been replaced by chronic diseases. These include the cancers, diabetes, and heart and lung diseases. Significantly, these conditions largely result from poor diet, tobacco and alcohol abuse and sedentary living. Cardiovascular disease is now the main cause of death in western nations.

Insulin resistance can precede the symptoms of syndrome X by many years. Early detection is therefore essential.

An editorial comment in the *British Medical Journal* in 2003 asked these questions:

> Could symptom causation be related to altered function without actual disease?
> Could disease causation be of greater significance and value for the patient than simply naming late-stage symptoms with the names of diseases?

The editorial proposed that the term 'functional illness' would be preferable and more acceptable to patients than 'medically unexplained symptoms'.

'Functional illness' serves to describe syndrome X very well. Such a diagnosis can exclude predictable diagnostic test results, and also actual damage or disease, in favour of a more functional definition – that organs and systems are inefficient.

Syndrome X – summary

Syndrome X, or the metabolic syndrome, is becoming a very common cause of CFS, involving insulin resistance, obesity, nutritional deficiencies and a risk of elevated blood pressure, coronary heart disease, diabetes, altered blood fats and hormones. I shall describe treatment strategies for the syndrome in chapter 6 (see page 226).

Diabetes

An important member of the family of blood sugar disorders is diabetes mellitus. There are two types: type I and type II. Fatigue is regularly seen as a symptom of both.

Type 1 is an acquired or inherited auto-immune illness in which the pancreas fails to provide sufficient insulin. Sufferers are usually 'insulin dependent', relying on regular injections.

Type II diabetes, also known as 'non-insulin-dependent diabetes mellitus' (NIDDM) is far more common, accounting for more than 90% of all diabetics. It has been called the 'prosperity disease' as it is so often linked with overeating processed foods, especially refined carbohydrates. Type II diabetes is virtually unknown in poorer countries. They are, however, catching up. An average of approximately 25% of people living in Europe and the USA are considered to be 'pre-diabetic'. The condition has also been termed 'late onset diabetes' because the symptoms often show in those aged 60+. Unfortunately it is increasingly being diagnosed in young people in their twenties, or even teens, and is reaching epidemic proportions in many western nations, in parallel with the current obesity epidemic.

Type II diabetes involves raised blood sugar levels, resulting from an inability to use insulin effectively (insulin resistance). Paradoxically the blood insulin can also be raised as the body attempts to compensate for the increasing resistance. Glucose intolerance, low blood sugar episodes, heart and blood circulation disorders and obesity are typical consequences, as is fatigue.

In addition to the clear association with over-processed, refined, high-carbohydrate diets that are nutrient deficient, excessive alcohol and a sedentary lifestyle also contribute. Significantly, up to 80% of type II diabetics are seriously overweight prior to their diagnosis.

Back in 1983 I wrote a book entitled *Diets to Help Diabetes*. At that time there was a growing obsession with the dangers of fat in our diet and the risks of high dietary cholesterol causing obesity and heart disease. It was assumed that an ideal diet for the overweight type II diabetic was low in fat and high in carbohydrates (though my book did not advocate this). Even then it was a mistaken view. Unfortunately, fat and protein intake in the West has reduced since the 1980s and carbohydrate consumption has increased, today being hidden behind the safety 'smoke screen' of high fibre and wholemeal preferences. All carbohydrate metabolism requires insulin; brown or white bread, or cereal, are only minimally different in their effect on blood glucose. In chapter 6 (see page 230) I shall discuss diabetic diets in some detail given the importance of controlling blood sugar levels in relieving fatigue.

Chapter summary

Readers may think that dwelling on the causes of CFS is unnecessary in this book, and that I should simply be discussing the symptoms and, perhaps most importantly, the treatment. In my experience, having treated CFS for over 40 years, I have learnt that the majority of patients wish to know why they feel the way they do and what has caused their problems.

I have attempted in this chapter to show that there may be diagnosable, physical causes to explain the distressing symptoms of CFS, but, as I have explained here, and elsewhere in this book, I do not accept that CFS can result from a single cause. Although it may be very helpful for a practitioner to be presented with a single cause to treat, this is very rare.

Many of the causes described in this chapter are interrelated. Let me offer an example: iron-deficient anaemia can depress thyroid function, which can render the adrenal system less efficient. This in turn can cause poor stress-handling and low blood sugar, all of which can contribute to chronic fatigue. Such a scenario highlights the need to view CFS as a group of possible symptoms with several overlapping causes.

Invariably with CFS patients, one or two dominant causes can be identified, and, of course, successful treatment of these causes can at times produce considerable symptom-relief. However, I find that it can be more rewarding to embrace the concept of multiple causes when diagnosing and subsequently treating the exhaustion so characteristic of CFS. Given the complexity of this condition, and its variation between individuals, it is only by taking the sufferer's detailed case-history and using specific individualised testing that the causes of CFS in a particular person can be discovered.

This chapter has focused on frequently seen causes of CFS. In the next chapter I will highlight other less frequently seen causes.

Chapter 4

Less common causes contributing to chronic fatigue syndrome

I have included this chapter, on less common contributory factors, to emphasise the complex nature of CFS causation. It is very doubtful that any one of these less frequently seen causes of fatigue leads to chronic exhaustion, but, as I have tried to stress throughout this book, in 40 years I have never seen a patient with a single, stand-alone cause for their CFS. No matter how obscure and trivial these factors may be, they still need to be identified, and if necessary included, within a successful treatment strategy for severe fatigue.

Drug side-effects

Pharmaceutical companies are obliged by law to test for drug safety and to identify and report on any side-effects their drugs may cause. This requirement applies to over-the-counter drugs as well as to prescription drugs. Unfortunately, the drug manufacturers are not called upon to report on side-effects that arise when drugs are prescribed in combination with several other drugs. I often see patients who are taking more than six, or even eight, different prescription drugs for a variety of symptoms and illnesses. As many drugs are prescribed to reduce acute symptoms (for example, infections, stress, pain), the commonest side-effects tend to include fatigue, digestive function symptoms and a general lowering of metabolic efficiency. An example of a drug that is commonly bought over-the-counter is **ibuprofen** (one of the many non-steroid anti-inflammatory drugs, or 'NSAIDs', which also include aspirin). The listed side-effects are as follows: gastro-intestinal discomfort, nausea and diarrhoea with occasional gastric or duodenal ulceration, rashes, headaches, nervousness, depression, insomnia, tinnitus, fatigue and occasionally severe exhaustion.

Another pain killer that is commonly self-prescribed, or prescribed by general practitioners, is **codeine phosphate**, which is an 'opioid analgesic'. Side-effects can include: nausea, vomiting, low blood pressure, vertigo, mood changes, dizziness, confusion, drowsiness, insomnia and many others.

The **ACE inhibitor drugs** (such as Captopril, Ramipril and Benazepril) are prescribed on a huge scale for high blood pressure. (In my experience, they are often over-prescribed as there is a tendency to lower the threshold of diagnosis). Side-effects include: low blood pressure, throat infections, sinusitis, nausea, vomiting, diarrhoea, abdominal pain, hypoglycaemia, headaches, dizziness, fatigue, taste disturbances, myalgia (muscle pain) and many others.

Propranolol hydrochloride is prescribed as Inderal, Atenolol and other drugs for the treatment of angina, heart rhythm conditions, high blood pressure and various other illnesses. Grouped under the heading of **beta-blockers**, their side-effects can include: low blood pressure, digestive disturbances, dyspnoea (breathlessness), headaches, insomnia, fatigue, dizziness, vertigo, visual problems, alopecia (hair loss) and various rashes.

A very controversial family of drugs, being increasingly prescribed to reduce cholesterol levels, are the **statins**. We are persuaded to believe that raised cholesterol is a major cause of heart disease and any drug that lowers cholesterol must therefore be a life-saver. The definition of 'abnormal' cholesterol seems to be constantly changing; increasingly lower thresholds are being recommended to define what constitutes high cholesterol. More details of cholesterol tests and interpretation follow later in the book but to quote from my earlier book *Why Am I So Tired?* in which I describe the treatment of thyroid disorders, I make the following observations regarding cholesterol: 'It is a fat-soluble, steroid alcohol, found chiefly in animal fats, oils and egg yolk. It is widely distributed in the body, being found chiefly in the bile, blood, brain tissue, the liver and kidneys. Also the adrenal glands and the fatty casing of nerves. Its many functions include fatty acid transport and absorption and the synthesis of vitamin D on the skin's surface. It also acts as an essential precursor for the adrenal hormones (cortisol, DHEA, aldosterone, etc) and the sex hormones (progesterone, oestrogen and testosterone). It is worth noting that around 80% of the cholesterol in our blood is synthesised directly by the liver and only 20% has a dietary source. Trials have confirmed that when cholesterol-free diets have been followed for several weeks, the blood cholesterol has actually risen as a result of its increased production by the liver.'

Whatever your view of the cholesterol theory, there is no question that statins cause fatigue. To quote an article in the *Daily Mail* (12 June 2012), 'The energy-sapping effect of taking statins is greater than previously thought. Women taking the anti-cholesterol drugs are particularly at risk of fatigue. Two in five women patients had less energy than before; with one in 10 saying they felt "much worse".' Studies have shown that statins inhibit the synthesis of the micro-nutrient 'co-enzyme Q-10' (also known as 'ubiquinone'). This is a component of our energy production in the mitrochondria of all the body's cells. The heart muscle in particular depends on co-enzyme Q-10. There is now a trend for many cardiologists to prescribe co-enzyme Q-10 with statins.

The Medicines and Healthcare Regulatory Products Agency has warned about the additional risks of sleep disturbance, memory loss and depression with statins. However, perhaps the most serious side-effect, aside from fatigue, is myalgia (muscle pain); muscle tenderness and weakness can also result. Readers will be aware that such side-effects closely parallel the symptoms of fibromyalgia. Numbness of the hands and feet, with pain, headaches and loss of appetite, are also typical statin side-effects.

Many other drugs can cause fatigued sufferers to feel worse. The liver is our chief detoxing organ and many drugs can stress the liver and worsen symptoms.

Anti-depressants
Anti-depressants have been termed the pharmaceutical 'golden goose'. Sales run into tens of millions of pounds. Fatigue and drowsiness are typical side-effects, as are nausea, vomiting, abdominal pain, diarrhoea and constipation,

muscle and joint pain, anxiety, insomnia, tremor, dizziness and suicidal tendencies. Unfortunately, these drugs are not only prescribed for 'clinical depression'. They are increasingly being recommended for aches and pains, such as backache and sciatica. The American Psychiatric Association has recently defined bereavement as a 'major depressive disorder', when sadness, weeping and poor concentration last longer than two weeks! This means more prescriptions and more profits for the drug companies.

Chronic infections and CFS

The role of infections as a contributory cause of chronic fatigue is a disputed subject. We are all aware of the hang-over effect resulting from a bout of 'flu or even a heavy cold. The immune system can become exhausted with chronic infections. The question that is so difficult to answer is, 'To what extent do chronic infections contribute to CFS?' Is symptom severity and duration closely linked to the infection or to a patient's immune efficiency? With epidemics there are always survivors. I list below some chronic infections which have an important link with CFS.

Epstein-Barr virus (EBV) – Also known as glandular fever or 'kissing disease', the main symptom of Epstein-Barr vius is fatigue. This virus can be identified with a blood test, including both previous and current infections.

Lyme disease (Borreliosis) – One of a large family of diseases transmitted by ticks, Lyme disease is caused by the *Borrelia burgdorferi* bacteria. The bacteria live in ticks that in turn live on deer, sheep, hedgehogs and other warm-blooded creatures, including birds, and there is evidence that pets can also carry the infection. The disease was identified in 1975 after an epidemic occurred in the town of Old Lyme in Connecticut, USA, giving it its name. It was known, however, in Victorian times. High risk areas in the UK include Exmoor, the New Forest, the Scottish Highlands and the Lake District, along with the North York moors and the South Downs. Early symptoms include a characteristic circular rash – this can measure six inches across – followed by 'flu-like symptoms. Long-term symptoms, if not diagnosed, can include fatigue and muscle and joint pain. There can be many other symptoms if it remains untreated, including blindness, paralysis, deafness and severe pain as Lyme disease can attack the central nervous system. The condition is difficult to diagnose. Blood testing can be inconclusive and antibiotic courses are not always successful. Lyme disease is thought to be the hidden source of many cases of undiagnosed CFS. Up to 10,000 cases annually have been suspected in the UK (*Daily Mail* 1 April 2008).

Cytomegalovirus (CMV) – Blood testing shows that up to 90% of adults have experienced CMV infection at some time prior to being tested. Fortunately, the infection is usually symptom-free. However, in children and pregnant women and those whose immune system efficiency has been compromised by organ transplants, immunosuppressant drugs or infections, symptoms can show. These are very similar to glandular fever, with fever and fatigue. With AIDS, CMV is the most common viral complication and can lead to blindness, liver damage or death. The pain in the affected nerves can persist for months after the infection ('post-herpetic neuralgia').

Chronic hepatitis – This can often result from an autoimmune reaction, sparked most commonly by the hepatitis C virus. Illegal drugs, the sharing of needles for injecting them, and alcoholism also contribute to the spread of hepatitis. Once again, the commonest symptom is fatigue, with loss of appetite, jaundice and abdominal discomfort. In young women, who are much more prone to hepatitis C than men, symptoms can include acne, cessation of periods, joint pain, thyroid and kidney inflammation and anaemia.

Environmental toxins

Toxic chemicals or 'xenobiotics' have been defined as 'chemical substances that are foreign and usually harmful to living organisms'. Xenobiotics are also known as POPS ('persistent organic pollutants'). Many POPS in our environment are cancer forming. They are known to cause immune system and thyroid disruption and behavioural problems in children. Rachel Carson's important book *Silent Spring*, published in 1962, was probably the first nontechnical book to make the public aware of environmental poisons. POPS can take up to 100 years to bio-degrade. Since World War II, it has been estimated that more than 80,000 such chemicals have entered the environment.

A call for a ban on 11 of the 'dirty dozen' top pollutants (see table 2.1) was recommended in 2001 by the United Nations Environment Programme. A good example of the 'stable-door' concept – as outlined above, many POPS degrade very slowly over a century.

Table 2.1: POPS – The environment and dietary sources of persistent organic pollutants: the 'dirty dozen'

Type	Sources – Environmental	Sources – Dietary
Dioxins, Furans	By-products of petroleum industry and chlorine bleaching in pulp and paper mills; hospital and council incinerators	Meat, poultry, dairy products, trout, salmon, water fowl, deer, muskrat, moose etc
PCBs	'Fire resistant' synthetic products made before 1977; old electrical equipment; leaky containers in PCB disposal sites	Great Lakes fish (eg lake trout, salmon), Arctic marine mammals, breast milk
Aldrin	Pesticide used against insects in the soil to protect crops such as corn and potatoes	Dairy products, meat, fish, oils and fats, potatoes and root vegetables
Chlordane	Broad spectrum contact insecticide used on vegetables, grains, maize, oilseed, potatoes, sugar cane, beets, fruits, nuts, cotton and jute	Use has been severely restricted so food does not appear to be a major pathway of exposure now; air may be a pathway because of continued use as termite control (in the USA)
DDT	Pesticide widely used during World War II to protect soldiers and civilians against diseases spread by insects	Fish, dairy products, fat of cattle, hogs, poultry and sheep, eggs, vegetables, breast milk
Dieldrin	Insecticide used to control insects in soil	Same as aldrin
Endrin	Foliar (leaf) insecticide used on field crops such as cotton	Current dietary exposure thought to be minimal because of restricted use

continued

Heptachlor	Non-systemic stomach and contact insecticide used to control insects in soil	Detected in the blood of US and Australian cattle in 1990; current dietary exposure thought to be minimal because of restricted use
HCB	Fungicide used for seed treatment	HCB-treated grain; current dietary exposure thought to be low because of severely restricted use
Mirex	Stomach (as opposed to 'contact') insecticide used to control ants, termites and mealy bugs	Meat, fish, wild game, marine bird eggs, sea mammals
Toxaphene	Contact insecticide used primarily on cotton, cereal, grains, fruits, nuts and vegetables and used to control ticks and mites in livestock	Dietary exposure thought to be very low because of restricted use; however, there is a local problem with some fish in Lake Superior, USA

Key: PCBs - polychlorinated biphenyls; DDT - dichloro-diphenyltrichloroethane; HCB - hexachlorobenzene
Source: Contaminant profiles. In: *Health and the Environment. The Health and Environment Handbook for Health Professionals.* Ottawa: Health Canada 1998.

Many activities and employments involve contact with chemicals that can trigger or exacerbate CFS. To indicate the great variety of possible contacts I include the sample lists below.

Possible pesticide contacts

Many types of plant sprays, including those used on farms and in market gardens, domestic gardens and greenhouses, contain pesticides. Animal treatments, including chicken farm fumigation, sheep dips, and dog, cat and cattle parasite treatments also contain them. Examples of occupational exposure include agricultural spray contact by those who deliver pesticides to farms, as well as the farmers themselves, and those who work in sheep markets; also people working with timber in houses and factories.

Domestic poisons

Un-burnt hydrocarbons

On a domestic level there are many poisons in our environment. One of the most important to be aware of are un-burnt hydrocarbons. These are organic compounds consisting of carbon and hydrogen and are by-products of oil, coal, gas and wood burning. Examples include benzene, toluene and naphalene with chlorine substitution. The chlorinated hydrocarbons are used in industrial solvents, refrigerators and dry cleaning fluids, also chloroform. Other hydrocarbons include methane, propane and the butanes. A further group include ethylene, propylene, acetylene and again the butanes. Although with gas fires and heaters the cause of poisoning and even death is usually attributed to carbon monoxide, long-term poisoning with un-burnt hydrocarbons can cause chronic fatigue.

Other domestic environmental poisoning agents that contribute to CFS include glues, paints, disinfectants, bleaches, carpet solvents, and cosmetic dyes, especially those used for hair colouring.

The controversial 'sick building' syndrome is thought by many to result from the solvents in new carpets, particularly exacerbated by poor ventilation. Low-frequency sound (see below) from poorly installed air conditioning systems can also contribute to the symptoms.

Carbon monoxide poisoning

A frequently underestimated cause of CFS is low levels of domestic carbon monoxide (CO). The gas is tasteless, colourless and odourless. The levels of gas in a house can build up over many months, often resulting from a chimney blockage or faulty, inefficient ventilation. It can be produced when fossil fuels do not completely burn.

Symptoms of chronic CO poisoning are frequently diagnosed as viral, as they can include unexplained fatigue, headaches, nausea, palpitations, dizziness, chest pains, hearing loss and poor memory. A significant diagnostic clue to the poisoning is the reduction of symptoms when away from the home environment. The advice frequently offered, 'Go home and rest', can therefore be fatally inappropriate.

The gas becomes lethal by replacing the oxygen in our blood. Carbon monoxide is around 200 times more likely to bind to haemoglobin than is oxygen. Hence our major organs can become oxygen deficient. Heart failure and/or brain damage and coma can result, even death.

The average death toll from CO poisoning in the UK is approximately 40-50 persons each year. However, it is thought likely that many more suffer the symptoms of a long-term gradual gas build-up. The problem is not always diagnosed, unless CO poisoning is suspected by the police or Coroner. Fortunately, inexpensive and effective audible carbon monoxide sensors or detectors for wall mounting can be bought from most ironmongers and DIY stores. These are a very worthwhile investment, particularly if children or the elderly (who perhaps rarely leave the house) live in a house with any fuel-burning appliances.

Multiple-chemical sensitivity syndromes (MCSS)

Multiple-chemical sensitivity syndrome defines a disorder, very often causing chronic fatigue, that is triggered by low-level exposure to multiple chemical substances that are commonly found in our environment. It has been estimated that up to 40% of people suffering from CFS and 16% of fibromyalgia sufferers have MCSS. As with many fatigue conditions, it is more frequently found in women than in men.

Although the fatigue resulting from MCSS can be caused by many diverse triggers, the following list includes the most common:

Alcohol
Caffeine
Carpet and furniture odours
Drugs, various (legal and illegal)
Food additives
Nicotine
Painting materials
Perfumes and other cosmetics
Pesticides and herbicides
Sterilisers and cleaning agents
Vehicle exhaust fumes.

The controversy that surrounds MCSS is largely due to the question, 'Are these factors the cause of CFS symptoms or merely contributory?' Certainly, it is not unusual to identify several possible triggers from the above list in the environment of many patients. Pre-existing health problems, coupled with an inefficient immune system, are likely to make some people more vulnerable to MCSS.

Low-frequency sound (LFS) – 'the wind farm effect'

The critics of wind farms have focused their objections to the wind turbines on the areas of cost, environmental damage and the regulation of acceptable noise levels. Wildlife deaths from the wind turbines are also included in the debate. Recent Spanish government research confirms that each turbine kills on average 300 birds annually and an equal number of bats.

The symptoms experienced by those who live close to wind turbines include: insomnia, fatigue, anxiety, dizziness, headaches, mood swings, nausea, depression, palpitations, raised blood pressure, poor memory, tinnitus and poor concentration. Many of these symptoms are a result of low-frequency sound, or 'infra-sound', produced by wind turbines.

The American physiologist Alec Salt has studied the subject for 40 years and has stated, 'The idea that there is no problem with infra-sound couldn't be more wrong; the responses of the human ear to low-frequency sound are just enormous. Bigger than anything in the audible range.' It has been known for over 20 years that the transmission of infra-sound creates many biophysical effects. These can include nausea, vomiting and disorientation. Wind farms have been described as, 'The greatest political blunder of our time and the biggest health scandal of our age.'

A clear relationship has been established between wind farms and the health of those living close to the turbines. Those being put up now are more than double the size of those erected 15 years ago and there are currently 4,000 turbines in the UK; many more are planned.

Aero-toxic syndrome

This rather sinister title describes symptoms caused by breathing contaminated air in jet aircraft. A frequent explanation for this syndrome is 'jet lag', that is thought to be caused by crossing time zones, which is known to weaken the immune system. Aero-toxic symptoms are in fact caused by inhaling toxic oil components and derivatives. With short-term exposures, the effects and subsequent symptoms are brief and reversible. However, repeated or prolonged exposures, as can be experienced in long flights, can cause severe symptoms. Many prematurely retired air crew who have left their jobs on medical grounds suffer inexplicable neurological symptoms.

What are known as 'fume events' result from all the air within a jet aircraft originating from the engines. This is known as 'bleed air' and this air comes from the section of the engine which needs frequent lubrication. Any leaking oil mixes with the very hot bleed air to create fumes and/or smoke. Jet aircraft need to use synthetic chemicals for lubrication, which contain organophosphate additives. The oil can also be partially decomposed. The contamination within the passenger compartment therefore consists chiefly of a combination of the oil fumes, the additives and the decomposition products.

The symptoms of the aero-toxic syndrome can include: fatigue, tremors, nausea, diarrhoea, vomiting, confusion, poor memory, coughs and chest restriction, vertigo, tinnitus, general confusion and poor concentration; nose and eye irritation and palpitations, insomnia, depression and anxiety have also been noted. This phenomenon should be considered as a cause of fatigue in frequent travellers.

Toxic metals

Chronic fatigue is a common symptom of toxic metal exposure. This section can only be a summary of what is a vast subject. Safety thresholds with many toxic metals have yet to be established. However, it has long been suspected that even trace amounts of some of the toxic metals can cause symptoms.

Any chemicals that are foreign to human metabolism are termed 'xenobiotics' (see 'Toxic chemicals' earlier in this chapter – page 75). For now I shall simply list the toxic metals and outline possible sources and the symptoms they can cause. Iron is not classed as 'toxic', but in excessive amounts ('haemochromatosis' – see page 85) it can be a source of many symptoms and it is therefore included in this section of the book. Copper is included for the same reason.

The toxic metals include: aluminium, arsenic, cadmium, copper, lead, manganese, mercury and nickel. People with multiple symptoms and chronic fatigue are often advised to have tests to screen for any toxic metal burden. Such testing can be with hair analysis, blood profiles or urine analysis. The majority of laboratories offer such tests. Unfortunately, many blood tests do not indicate tissue levels of toxic metals and as biopsies are impractical and costly, urine testing is often seen as the most reliable method to assess a toxic metal build up. This can often result from low-level but long-term exposure.

As I describe more fully below, toxic metals have many sources. These include: environmental (rural and urban), occupational, dietary, pharmaceutical (prescription and over-the-counter drugs), cosmetics, plant medicines, exhaust fumes, tobacco and contact with metals in jewellery. The influence of the mercury amalgam used in dental work is described after this section. I believe that it deserves special mention.

Sources and typical symptoms of metal toxicity
Aluminium (Al)
As with many other toxic metals, the absorption of aluminium can be enhanced by increased gut permeability (leaky gut syndrome). Moreover, in iron-deficient anaemia, aluminium uptake is also increased. Calcium and magnesium deficiency can also have this effect.

Sources – Many food stuffs contain aluminium, and tap water may contain aluminium fluoride. Aluminium cooking vessels and aluminium foil are also sources of this metal. Various over-the-counter analgesics and antacids contain aluminium, as do anti-sweating remedies and nearly all deodorants. Traces are also found in various types of cosmetics. Exhaust fumes and tobacco smoke are also on the list.

Symptoms – As aluminium excess can build up in the brain, it is a suspected factor contributing to Alzheimer's disease and motor neurone disease; also to seizures, behavioural disorders, memory loss, other types of dementia, headaches, fatigue, epilepsy, tremors and even paralysis and death. All of these symptoms have been observed. In addition, digestive disorders, abdominal colic, gastritis, rashes, insomnia, cramp, infertility and high blood pressure are typical symptoms caused by an excess of aluminium.

Arsenic (As)

Sources – Listed as the 'Number 1' toxin by the American Agency for Toxic Substances and Disease Registration, although it is rare to see its harmful effects, arsenic is usually one of the metals that laboratories list under 'occupational health-trace metals'. Other than industrial sources, its chief sources are garden sprays and wallpapers. It may also be contained in weed killers, insecticides and herbicides. Water and wine can also be contaminated.

Symptoms – Arsenic can seriously compromise the production of energy in any organ or system. Symptoms are therefore widespread, including fatigue, paraesthesia (numbness) in limbs, headaches, skin conditions, seizures, kidney and liver disorders, muscle weakness and hair loss. It can also cause a rare form of liver cancer. Extreme fear and anxiety with suicidal thoughts have also been noted as a result of arsenic poisoning.

Cadmium (Cd)

Sources – Possibly the chief sources of cadmium exposure are from exhaust fumes and tobacco smoke. The metal gives off a characteristic onion/garlic odour. Excessive levels of cadmium can also result from zinc deficiency as normally zinc competes with cadmium to keep levels low. Cadmium-plated bolts, nuts and screws give off the metal if heated, sanded or power buffed. Other sources include coal-burning units, certain paints, fungicides and pesticides, and it can also be present in many fish, organ meats and coffee.

Symptoms – With accumulated exposure, symptoms can include: fatigue, anaemia, poor immunity, emphysema, zinc deficiency with resulting slow healing, hair loss, weight loss, nausea, headaches, colic, vomiting, diarrhoea and high blood pressure. Behavioural problems, difficulties with learning, poor memory and irrational anxiety and irritability are also possible symptoms. There can be a very gradual onset of symptoms and cadmium is often overlooked as a cause.

Copper (Cu)

Sources – Any copper not bound to a protein in our food is potentially toxic. Unbound copper can result from acid food or drink in prolonged contact with copper vessels. Excess copper consumption is itself rare. The chief source of copper toxicity, in households in particular, is copper pans, piping and water heaters. Such toxicity is worse with acid water. Food sources include various canned greens, where copper is added to increase the colour, soya beans and some meats (copper sulphate is included in animal feedstuffs as a growth enhancer). Other sources include certain prescription drugs – for example, the contraceptive pill. Tobacco and zinc-deficiency can also elevate copper to excess.

Wilson's disease – This is a rare hereditary condition that results from the liver's inability to excrete any excess copper. As a result, there is a build-up of copper in the liver, causing actual damage. Copper is released directly into the blood stream and into the brain and eyes. Symptoms can show at around five years of age and indicate brain damage – for example, tremors, poor coordination and personality changes. If there is a family history of Wilson's disease, tests should be performed on children aged two years.

Symptoms – Unbound copper consumed even in small amounts can cause fatigue, nausea, diarrhoea and vomiting. Also low blood sugar, headaches, anaemia, hair loss, pre-menstrual syndrome, rashes, indigestion and, if the poisoning is severe, the liver and kidneys can be damaged. Children can develop ADHD (attention-deficit hyperactivity disorder) or hyperactivity, autism and infections.

Lead (Pb)

Sources – The adverse effects of various toxic metals have been identified (usually retrospectively) by studying repeated household contact or industrial use. An obvious example is the suspicion that the lead-based drinking vessels regularly used by the wealthy ruling Romans contributed to the eventual fall of the Roman Empire. The list of symptoms below will explain how this might have happened. The Roman aqueducts were lined with lead and, as lead acetate is sweet tasting, it was routinely added to Roman wine, for flavouring. Lead poisoning is also known to have been widespread in the 18th and 19th centuries in England, caused by rum and port being manufactured in lead vessels. The effects of exposure to toxic metals in such drinks, and later in industry, have been an important source of harmful side-effects. Even now, this problem arises. A report published in 1997 (*Lead and Public Health – the Dangers for Children*) by Eric Millstone stated that levels of lead in British drinking water were 'dangerously high', the chief source being lead pipes. He estimated that one in 10 children suffered the effects of lead poisoning.

Symptoms – These include fatigue, diarrhoea and constipation, nausea and vomiting, headaches, thyroid malfunction, anaemia, cirrhosis of the liver, insomnia, ankle and wrist weakness, abdominal cramping, kidney damage, sterility, schizophrenia, aggressive behaviour, memory loss, nightmares, a metallic taste in the mouth and aching in muscles and joints. Truly a catalogue of symptoms.

Heavy metals

Toxic metals and heavy metals tend to be interchangeable terms, although 'toxic' is preferred. The use of 'heavy' is usually confined to the toxic metals with a high atomic weight. These include cadmium, lead, mercury, arsenic, thallium and antimony.

Haemochromatosis (iron overload)

Haemochromatosis is the grand-sounding name for a disorder that is characterised by an excessively high level of iron in the body. It is often overlooked or misinterpreted because of the wrong tests being chosen. Blood iron and haemoglobin levels can both be 'normal'. Diagnosis is based on two blood tests:

> **Ferritin** – A protein that stores iron, chiefly in the liver, spleen and bone-marrow
>
> **Transferrin** – Another protein that carries the iron that is not found inside the red blood cells

Although medical dictionaries and textbooks tend to describe haemochromatosis as a rare condition, I am currently seeing three patients with high ferritin levels. This suggests that it is not so obscure as to be ignored as yet another potential contributory cause of chronic fatigue.

Sources – High blood iron and ferritin can occur with excessive inappropriate blood transfusions or from taking too much supplementary iron over a prolonged period. However, the chief cause of this condition is genetic, being a hereditary disorder with the official medical name of 'primary haemochromatosis'.

Symptoms – These can initially be vague and with a gradual onset. In fact the time required to accumulate an excess level of blood iron and ferritin can be from three to 50 years. This time-scale serves to explain why the usual age at which symptoms appear in men can be 35–50 years. However, in women, the monthly menstrual blood loss usually ensures that the symptoms of inappropriate iron accumulation are delayed until the onset of menopause. For this reason, only approximately 10% of patients with the symptoms of haemochromatosis are female.

With many disorders and diseases, excessive under-activity and over-activity of a particular organ or function can give rise to very similar symptoms. This apparent contradiction applies to the symptoms of iron deficiency and iron overload. Initially symptoms are vague and widespread, chief among them being fatigue and (with iron overload) bronze-coloured skin. However, other common symptoms and disorders can include diabetes, arthritis, impotence and infertility in men; also hypothyroidism.

Mercury amalgam

It is unlikely that any subject has attracted more rancour and dispute within the medical and dental professions than the influence of mercury amalgam fillings on CFS. Many dentists, particularly in central London, recommend complete removal of mercury fillings as a treatment for CFS. Although I have spoken to 20–25 patients over the previous two to three years, who have spent thousands of pounds on this service, I have found very few who can report any relief of their symptoms. I know that it could be argued that those patients who benefit from such treatment would have little cause to consult me. However, I am not alone in viewing the mercury amalgam removal protocol as being difficult to prove and perhaps over-commercialised.

No doubt, many readers will wonder what all the fuss is about. There must surely be very few dental patients *without* mercury amalgam fillings.

Why is this routine dental treatment now being described as a health risk and a major cause of chronic fatigue? To answer that, we need to know what mercury amalgam is.

Mercury amalgam has been in use for around 190 years. It consists of a mixture of 50% liquid mercury and a powder containing the minerals copper, tin, nickel and zinc. The USA Dental Association claims that the combination of metals in the amalgam renders it 'non-toxic'. By contrast, the French government is currently considering a ban on the use of amalgam fillings.

This amalgam is now used in around 80% of fillings. It has been known for some time that the mercury content tends to be released as a vapour and within seven to eight years approximately 50% of the mercury content has been released into the patient's body. After 20 years, up to 80% will have been released. Unfortunately, several toxic metals, including mercury, compete with nutritional minerals in our body. Many dentists claim that this accounts for the huge diversity of symptoms caused by mercury amalgam. Perhaps not surprisingly, dental workers are statistically the unhealthiest profession, with high levels of tissue mercury and a high percentage of mental, emotional and physical symptoms when compared with other professions.

The introduction of an increased copper content in amalgam fillings during the 1970s has tended to speed up the release of mercury vapour. Many physicians and dentists blame this change for the increase in patients diagnosed with CFS over the last 30 years.

Mercury toxicity can cause many symptoms, the chief of these being fatigue, poor immune function and a decrease in thyroid and adrenal efficiency. The most frequently asked question when discussing the relationship between chronic fatigue and dental amalgam symptoms is, 'Why does this affect some people and not others?' The other obvious question is, 'What can be done about it, apart from complete removal of amalgam from my teeth?' Unfortunately, removal of amalgam fillings increases the amount of mercury in a patient's circulation for many months.

In a very comprehensive book entitled *Chronic Fatigue Syndrome – a treatment guide'* the authors, Verrillo and Gellman, say the following about mercury fillings: 'Do not have all your fillings removed to eliminate potential leakage of mercury. While mercury poisoning resembles CFIDS (Chronic Fatigue and Immune Dysfunction Syndrome) in many ways, the two should not be confused. Elimination of numerous fillings is expensive, laborious and thoroughly stressful, requiring use of anaesthetics and other chemical substances that may cause harmful effects to a compromised immune system.' They suggest hair-mineral analysis testing before considering amalgam filling removal to check if there actually is any evidence of elevated mercury levels. They conclude with the following statement: 'Be forewarned, that although mercury is certainly toxic, it is not likely that the small quantity of mercury that can leak from fillings will cause the myriad persevering symptoms of CFIDS. The small number of people with CFIDS who have had fillings removed have not reported improvement. A few felt worse for days to several weeks afterward because of the exhausting nature of extensive filling removal and replacement.' (The term CFIDS is a popular American version of CFS.) Significantly, the section that deals with mercury amalgam in their very comprehensive, 400-page book is barely a full page in length.

Diagnosis of mercury toxicity

Tests are available for mercury excess. These include blood tests and urine tests. Several laboratories provide panels or profiles for toxic metals that include mercury. Unfortunately, the blood and urine tests tend to show only ongoing exposure to toxic metals and bear very little relationship to actual levels within the body's tissues. For this reason, many regard hair-mineral analysis as being the most effective test to identify mercury excess. As an example of its worth, the levels of hair mercury are significantly higher in people with multiple sclerosis (MS) than in people without the condition.

To end this section on an historical note, in the 19th century, mercury compounds were used in hat making. Mercury poisoning is still referred to at times as the 'mad hatters' disease'. Exposure to mercury can cause aggressiveness, mood swings and anti-social behaviour. So hatters may not have actually been insane; the 'mad' reference may have denoted bad temper.

Magnesium deficiency

You may wonder why, with so many vitamins, minerals, proteins and other nutrients to choose from, I have assigned a complete section to the mineral magnesium. Its significance is its part in the health of the mitochondria in our cells. Dr Sarah Myhill in her book *Diagnosing and Treating CFS* states that, 'I actually now believe that a low red cell magnesium is a symptom of mitrochondrial failure'. She continues, 'I see low magnesium almost routinely in patients with fatigue symptoms.'

Up to 400 milligrams of magnesium daily are considered essential for mitrochondrial support. The mitochondria are the energy-generating units within all cells in the body, sometimes referred to as our 'cellular batteries'. It is not therefore surprising that CFS is seen by many physicians as an expression of mitochondrial failure. Over 300 different body enzymes are dependent on magnesium. Not surprisingly, the symptoms of deficiency are many and varied, though heart problems are the chief indicator. Unfortunately this mineral is virtually absent from American and European junk food diets. Modern soil also tends to be deficient in magnesium.

As I have discussed elsewhere in this book (see page 115), our blood tends to be given metabolic priority when minerals are in short supply. Testing for magnesium levels in whole blood (the preferred test choice) is for this reason of little diagnostic value. Blood levels are maintained at the expense of levels within the cells.

Dosages of magnesium orotate or glycinate in daily amounts of 500 to 1000 milligrams have been known to assist not only chronic fatigue, but also asthma, fibromyalgia, migraine, pre-menstrual syndrome, cramping, intermittent claudication (muscle pain during exercise) and DVT (deep vein thrombosis). It has also been prescribed for hypoglycaemia and mitral valve disorders. Intra-muscular injections of magnesium have in recent years become a fashionable treatment for CFS in London clinics. Although such treatment can provide symptom-relief, it is preferable if the magnesium is part of a total treatment supplement programme that is individually tailored for each patient.

Omega-6 and omega-3 deficiency

I wonder just how many of you understand the terms 'omega-3' and 'omega-6'. Perhaps I need to explain. They are terms for unsaturated fatty acids. The contents of omega-3 and omega-6 are as follows:

Omega-3 (W) – Derivatives
    Alpha-linolenic acid (LNA)
    Stearidonic acid (SDA)
    Eicosopentaenoic acid (EPA)
    Docosahexaenoic acid (DHA)

Omega-6 (W) – Derivatives
    Linolenic acid (LA)
    Gamma-linolenic acid (GLA)
    Arachidonic acid (AA)

Two members of the omega-3 and -6 families are what are termed 'essential fatty acids'; that is for the simple reason that our bodies cannot manufacture then and they must therefore be sourced from what we eat and drink. These are:

    Linoleic acid (LA) (omega-6)
    Alpha-linolenic acid (LNA) (omega-3)

LNA is found in flaxseed oil, hemp, walnut oil, rape (canola), soybean oil, cold water fish, game and eggs. Unfortunately, the best food sources of LNA have become either expensive to buy, and so are rarely consumed, or are badly prepared and cooked and therefore regarded as 'unhealthy'. Fish has become an expensive protein on a par with steak, hence its reduced availability and consumption. When my wife shops at our local French country markets, she finds that most of the fish tends to be more costly than quality beef.

It is unfortunate that the name of a major group of essential nutrients – fats – is also used to describe being overweight. The fats have acquired a bad reputation that tends to link their consumption with obesity. There are, however, some fats that we must obtain from our food in order to maintain good health. In a classic book entitled *Chronic Fatigue Syndrome – a natural way to treat CFS/ME*, the author, Professor Basant K Puri, writes, 'I came to the conclusion that one of the key components needed to treat Chronic Fatigue Syndrome is a combination of ultra-pure EPA (omega-3) free of any DHA and virgin evening primrose oil (omega-6).' Dr Robert Atkins, an American nutrition doctor and author of the famous *Atkins Diet* books, has stated that, 'What is becoming inescapably clear is that the essential fatty acids are collectively the number one missing ingredient in the American diet.'

The medical and hence the public view is to regard all fats as dangerous. It is believed that fats are the chief cause of heart disease, cancer, diabetes, obesity and a wide range of other health problems. Consequently, consumption of omega-3 fats has reduced. Meanwhile, the obsession with the health benefits of evening primrose oil (omega-6) has contributed to a situation where the ratio of omega-3 to omega-6 in our diets has become seriously imbalanced in favour of omega-6.

The extract below from the Doctors Laboratory's laboratory guide is of interest. It describes an omega-3 to omega-6 blood test ratio.

Omega-3 fats are used as the building blocks for fat derived hormones such as prostaglandins and leukotrienes. The hormones with an omega-3 base tend to reduce inflammation, while those that have an omega-6 base increase inflammation. In the cell membrane the competition between these two essential fats has a direct bearing on the type of local hormone produced and the level of inflammation in the cell.

The omega-6 to omega-3 ratio in the cell membranes is key to the development of inflammatory disorders such as rheumatoid arthritis and heart disease.

Diets low in oily fish and high in grains will promote inflammation and affect good health. The ratio of omega-6 to omega-3 in the West is around 15 to 1, fifteen times more omega-6 on the cell membrane, promoting inflammation.

Having twice as much omega-6 is considered by most experts to be the optimal amount but a ratio of 2:1 is not easy to produce by diet alone. Many people are aware of the health benefits of omega-3 but the supplementation to achieve optimal health is erratic. Being able to test for Essential Red Cell Fatty Acids (the omega-6/omega-3 ratio) identifies a person's current status and is sufficiently specific to allow an accurate supplementation recommendation to be made.

Results show the Omega Ratio with a clear recommendation for the required level of omega supplementation (if any) to achieve optimal levels.

Insomnia

Insomnia is a major health problem and a widespread contributor to chronic fatigue. Unfortunately many insomniacs take a magic 'pill' to cure their problem instead of seeking and treating the cause or causes of their problem.

The generally held view is that we all need at least eight hours sleep each night. There are those who can become very distressed and anxious if this target is not reached. People aged 55–60 years may in fact only need five to six hours sleep each night, coupled with perhaps a brief siesta during the day. If a person complains that they cannot get to sleep until after midnight yet they feel normally vital on rising, it may well be that five to six hours sleep is sufficient for them. Regrettably it cannot be assumed that feeling tired on waking confirms a diagnosis of insomnia with insufficient sleep. As described elsewhere in this book, our blood sugar status, adrenal efficiency and other factors play important parts in influencing how we feel on rising. The night fast is a problem for many, whose metabolism, for various reasons, cannot sustain a normal blood sugar level throughout the night. My patients often report that if they avoid food for more than three or four hours during the day, they can feel tired and shaky, indicating an inappropriate lowering of their blood sugar level. Yet the same people may well be avoiding food for 12 hours or more through every night. It is not then surprising that they can wake with a headache, drowsiness and irritability. Some weight loss diets have advocated the 'no breakfast plan', which only worsens this tendency, by lengthening the night fast.

Causes of insomnia
Insomnia can be defined as an inability to fall asleep or a difficulty in returning to sleep after premature awakening. The principal causes are outlined below.

Sleep apnoea syndromes
Although there are several types of sleep apnoea, they are all caused by transient oxygen deprivation, as a result of the person stopping breathing. Typical symptoms include fatigue with sleepiness, irritability and headaches on rising, sluggish thinking and poor concentration, with reduced libido. Treatment recommendations are chiefly common-sense measures, such as

weight loss, quitting smoking, and avoiding anti-histamine sleep-aid drugs, such as Nytol. (These can unpredictable side-effects such as restlessness, agitation and nervousness.)

More severe forms of sleep apnoea may need specialised nocturnal dental appliances to facilitate easier breathing, or a nocturnal face mask to assist breathing. Oxygen delivery by nasal inserts can also be recommended. The oxygen level in the blood can be measured with an electrode in the finger or ear lobe. In really extreme cases, surgery may be recommended. Recognising and treating food intolerances has been known to relieve sleep apnoea.

Stress
Stress can cause physical tension. Any form of stress has the potential to cause adrenal fatigue and possible low blood sugar. Many people suffer stress through the night; sleep does not guarantee relaxation.

Caffeine
Excessive coffee drinking can rev-up the metabolism. Coffee is best drunk on waking and not on retiring.

Late meals
A small protein snack upon retiring for the night will assist the blood sugar but a heavy meal can cause sleep problems.

Erratic sleeping habits
Our metabolism thrives on routine to achieve a regular pattern for sleep onset and duration. It can therefore be helpful to have a routine bed-time and awakening.

Ventilation
A badly ventilated bedroom may lead to insufficient oxygen being available, resulting in sleeplessness.

Obesity (Obesity-hypoventilation syndrome)
For readers who are Charles Dickens's fans, this is also known as 'Pickwick syndrome'. Excessive body fat can reduce the flexibility of the chest, thus

reducing the volume of air reaching the lungs. If the excess fat is around the throat or below the diaphragm the air flow is further reduced.

Other causes of insomnia
I have covered the main causes of insomnia. There are, however, many other contributory causes of insufficient or disturbed sleep. These can include:

Muscle/joint pain, often worse with rest
Smoking and alcohol
Magnesium deficiency causing night cramps
Too much light at night can disturb the pineal gland that releases
       nature's sleep hormone, melatonin
Excessive TV and computer viewing before retiring: a recent study
       showed that computer screen light obstructs melatonin production
Excessive salt in food
Respiratory problems including asthma, allergic rhinitis, chronic
       catarrh, pleurisy, bronchitis and emphysema
Restless leg syndrome
Sleep phobia and nightmares
Recreational drug use
Mouth breathing resulting from nasal congestion
Menopausal hot-flushes with night sweats
Diabetic 'hypos' causing night sweats and restlessness
Poor quality mattress – 'Orthopaedic' mattresses can be too hard. A
       suitable double mattress needs to be a least 1000 spring composition
Many vitamin and mineral deficiencies can contribute to insomnia.

Dehydration

The suggestion that dehydration (water shortage) may be a contributory cause of fatigue will seem strange and unlikely to many readers. However, it is worth knowing that our bodies are composed of 25% solid matter and 75% water. In fact, brain tissue consists of around 85% water.

We tend to assume that as water is freely available, our bodies cannot be in short supply. This unfortunately is far from the truth. In

Dr F Batmanghelidj's excellent book *Your Body's Many Cries For Water*, he states that 75% of people are chronically dehydrated and the main trigger for daytime fatigue is lack of water. He further states that, 'unintentional chronic dehydration is at the root of many serious diseases, including asthma, renal dysfunction, endocrine system imbalance and adrenal fatigue, high blood pressure and other cardiovascular problems, arthritis, ulcers, pancreatitis, digestion difficulties and lower back pain.' He claims that to remain healthy we must drink approximately a full 8 ounce glass of pure water (preferably *not* tap water) every hour each day. Dehydration causes stress and stress causes further dehydration. Hence a vicious circle tends to be established.

A well-publicised case of death by dehydration recently involved a 22-year-old patient at one of the UK's top teaching hospital (St George's Hospital, Tooting, London). It was widely reported in July 2012, with suggestions of nursing incompetence, and wider fears about poor patient care in British hospitals. There are 300,000 largely untrained healthcare assistants in NHS hospitals, while there have been reports of hospital patients drinking the water from flower vases in their desperate need for fluids.

Even moderate dehydration can cause a dry mouth and tongue, with headache, dizziness on standing, pressure sores with prolonged bed rest, falls as a result of low blood pressure, and mental confusion. It can also lead to urinary tract infections and blood clotting resulting from blood thickening. Severe dehydration symptoms can include mental confusion, nausea, vomiting and acute kidney injury or failure. Dehydration can be a contributory cause of chronic fatigue, as well as other symptoms.

Histamine intolerance (HIT)

Histamine is a chemical produced from the protein histadine and it is present in all body tissues, its highest concentration being in the lungs. Histamine has various functions. These include: responding to inflammation by increasing the local blood supply, resulting in capillary dilation; contraction of smooth muscle tissue; influencing the secretion of acid and other substances in the stomach; and the acceleration of the heart rate as needed.

Histamine is normally metabolised and processed by an enzyme called 'diamine oxidase' (DAO), which is produced in the lining of the gut. Histadine chiefly enters our body via histamine-rich foods, including spinach, aubergine, pickles, cured meats, avocado, mature cheeses, yeast and tomatoes. There are various factors that can reduce the effectiveness of the vital DAO. These include local infections in the intestine, a course of antibiotics, certain drugs (particularly anaesthetics), food intolerances and alcohol. There are also various control systems in place to prevent histamine levels rising too high in the blood. However, any of the above factors can compromise this balance and the histamine level can rise. As with most intolerances, HIT results from a faulty metabolism that does not allow histamine to be properly metabolised.

Significantly, the symptoms of HIT include: indigestion, headaches, rhinitis, insomnia and fatigue. The fatigue is often worse after meals and on rising. Poor concentration, skin conditions, asthma, low blood pressure and body coldness are also common symptoms. Many of these symptoms are typical of CFS. (See *What HIT me?* by G Masterman, listed in Further reading.)

Nitrous oxide poisoning ('laughing gas')

Nitrous oxide is an anaesthetic gas and it has a legitimate use in surgery, though there are safer and equally effective substitutes. It is a commonly used dental anaesthetic and is also routinely used in caesarean sections and many other operations. It is used to sedate patients and provide pain relief. It is also a recreational drug, as it produces a sense of euphoria and a pleasant dreamlike state. Unfortunately, it can also inactivate vitamin B-12 and destroy vitamin B-12 stores. Those patients who unknowingly have a borderline B-12 deficiency are particularly vulnerable to neurological damage. Post-surgical B-12 deficiency is often blamed on the unavoidable side-effects of the surgery. It is not unusual to hear people say that they have not felt well since they underwent surgery, often with their new symptoms being quite unrelated to the reason for their operation. While this is blamed on the unavoidable effects of surgery, it may well be due in part to vitamin B-12 deficiency if the person concerned had a predisposing borderline problem at the outset.

The symptoms of post-operative reaction to nitrous oxide can include: fatigue, weakness, tremors, unsteady gait, depression, fibromyalgia, dementia, restless leg syndrome, vertigo, psychiatric disorders, weight loss and many other related symptoms.

The melatonin mystery

Communication within our nervous system is mediated by 'neurotransmitters' – chemicals that transmit signals from one nerve cell to the next. Melatonin is one of the neurotransmitters, and although it is prescribed for insomnia, recent research has shown that CFS sufferers tend to have too much when their blood is tested. It is thought that the higher levels of melatonin could be a result of an overstressed immune system owing to excessive stress or severe or repeated infections. Carbohydrates are known to increase melatonin levels, so this may present another sound reason to follow a low-carbohydrate diet.

Air pollution

London is the most polluted capital in Europe. Under EU directives all member states were obliged to bring pollution levels to safe medically-approved levels by 2010. Only three out of the 43 designated areas in the UK have succeeded. Air pollution kills thousands each year, including 4,300 in London.

Pollution is a major cause of asthma, particularly in children. There is currently an asthma epidemic in the UK which affects one in seven British children.

The concept of 'total load'

As with the previous chapter, you may view the possible causes listed in this chapter as bewildering and unlikely to be major influences on a person's health and vitality. However, bringing together the multiplicity of causes, large and small, is essential in understanding what the 'total load' may be for any individual CFS sufferer.

'Total load' describes the concept that a combination of various 'xenobiotics', or toxins, can together adversely influence our health. I believe that this paradigm can also be applied to CFS – while one factor alone may not be enough to make a person ill, it is the combination of factors and triggers that can lead to illness (see chapter 5).

The *Textbook of Functional Medicine* says, 'The concept of total load suggests that the totality of factors can seriously affect an individual's system of metabolic management.' I have discussed this notion with colleagues and medical doctors. There is general agreement with the view that CFS does not have a single cause, but many interrelated causes, all needing to be identified and treated. While it may at times be appropriate to give priority to perhaps one or two key causes, the 'total load' should always be considered and treated.

I appreciate that the many causes of CFS, and of illnesses generally, cannot always be successfully treated. This can particularly apply to environmental factors, domestic and employment stress and nutritional deficiencies that are linked perhaps to low income. Nevertheless, it is important to be aware of such factors, at least as a starting point for beneficial changes in your health.

Chapter 5

The diagnosis of chronic fatigue syndrome

In common with the many definitions and the great variety of treatments being offered to patients, the diagnosis of chronic fatigue is open to many different procedures and interpretations. This is particularly apparent when comparing the conventional medical perspective with the naturopathic view. I frequently remind my patients, when discussing their symptoms and treatment, that doctors 'do like a nice disease'. Perhaps this comment is a little flippant, but the fact remains that medical diagnosis is dependent on the need to identify, and, if possible, to give a name to a specific disease or malady, before treatment can begin. This protocol often results in chronically exhausted patients, who have perhaps suffered for several years, never being offered a meaningful diagnosis or an effective treatment.

Readers may ask, 'How can this happen?', the assumption being that a patient's symptoms can usually provide the diagnostic clues, supported by testing, to confirm the cause, or causes, of his/her health problem. Once a diagnosis has been established, then treatment can be prescribed. Unfortunately, patients' symptoms are no longer always seen as significant; test results often take precedence over the evaluation of symptoms, when a diagnosis is being considered.

With an area of ill-health as complex as chronic fatigue, I believe that it is essential to attempt to match the patients' symptoms with his/her test results. If you have CFS, this is what you should be looking for when finding a practitioner who can help you'. However, this is only feasible when:

1. The tests selected are relevant to the patient's symptom-picture and health history;

2. The subsequent interpretation of the test results accurately reflects the patient's symptom variety and severity.

This means taking a tailored approach to requesting and interpreting tests. I am told by many of my patients that they have had blood tests and then subsequently been informed that 'everything is normal'. This usually means that they have had a standard haematology and biochemistry blood test, which comprises 35–40 separate tests. These can include the blood cell counts (red and white), blood fats, liver function, blood sugar, proteins, uric acid (gout factor) and possibly thyroid function tests. But in diagnosis, one size does not fit all.

Test selection in diagnosis

Nutrition forms a very small part of European medical training. By far the largest part of the general practitioner's (GP's) training consists of learning about drug types and treatments. Very little emphasis is placed on life-style changes, diet or the use of nutritional supplements. Although correct test interpretation is an essential component of diagnosis, selecting the tests that will serve to reflect the individual is also vital. It is essential to recognise that there are variations in human body composition, nutritional status and needs, body chemistry and systems when deciding what tests are appropriate. Other important factors that influence selection include the person's gender, age, occupation, symptoms, health history, family health and, of course, past and current treatments. Assessing a person's health status and disease possibilities can be confused and often compromised when he/she is taking drugs to reduce or eliminate symptoms. Although no one likes to suffer pain, depression, exhaustion, indigestion or a range of debilitating symptoms, the symptoms themselves can provide very useful clues in arriving at a meaningful diagnosis.

Test selection for CFS

The basic screening profiles offered by the NHS and many private medical health insurance companies are rarely symptom related. They are usually requested to identify well-established health conditions, such as diabetes, anaemia, liver and gall bladder conditions, types of cancer, gout, kidney disease, heart disease and arthritis.

I currently send blood, saliva and urine samples to five different laboratories. Their total test selection amounts to over 2000 tests. I am not suggesting that any patient is likely to require 2000 tests. Many of these are costly, very specialised and often unnecessary. However, a personalised, specific test selection is of greater value for diagnosis than standardised hospital tests.

As far as I am aware, only the Acumen laboratory in the West of England offers specialised testing for fatigue. I shall outline test profiles later in this chapter.

You may ask, 'Just how do naturopaths test their patients?' This is a fair and justifiable question as naturopaths in the past have been criticised for being unscientific in their diagnostic approach. The word 'naturopathy' suggests natural and many readers still see 'natural cure' as being associated with fasting, enemas, hydrotherapy and vitamin supplements. I do have naturopathic colleagues who still regard blood testing as medical 'mumbo-jumbo', being misleading and pointless. Fortunately, such practitioners are in the minority, with a growing realisation within the profession that naturopaths need to work, where appropriate, alongside medical doctors, and not attempt to replace them. Regrettably, even in the 21st century, naturopathic diagnosis remains a rarely discussed subject. However, such groups as the Institute for Functional Medicine based in the USA are leading the way in a science-based healthcare approach, in particular providing functional, nutritional support for CFS patients. I shall discuss this further in chapter 6 (see page 168).

In addition to what and how tests are selected, just what are the differences when comparing GPs' tests with a naturopath's tests? How past and current results are interpreted serves to highlight the differences in procedure. Standard hospital and GP tests do not always have the subtlety to answer questions for patients with CFS. They *should* be able to identify such problems as anaemia, hypothyroidism, heart disease, diabetes and other serious conditions (though you will see later in this chapter that there are problems with both anaemia and hypothyroidism), but even so, I do see patients who have never had a blood test, or whose test results are very out of date, being perhaps five to 10 years old and diagnostically useless.

Test interpretation in diagnosis

You would be forgiven if you assumed that the normal ranges, as defined for specific blood test results, are standardised throughout the medical world, such a system being the essential basis for the precise diagnosis of any health problem. Unfortunately, this is not the case. Normal ranges are not standardised, let alone adjusted on a systematic basis for individual patients. The normal ranges for blood tests that are designed to identify diabetes, anaemia, cholesterol status, thyroid and adrenal function, for example, are just a few examples of the very different ranges defined as 'normal' by the various laboratories in different countries. Even within the UK there is great variation in the recommended normal ranges for many test results.

According to a recent book on the subject of faulty diagnosis (*Over Diagnosed* by Dr H Gilbert Welch *et al*), 'There is no scientific method or mathematical equation that will result in a single answer to the question of what should be defined as normal.' The authors maintain that, 'The medical community is engaged in a relentless drive to narrow that definition.'

Although over-diagnosis in the USA (which is often motivated by commercial priorities) is on the increase, the opposite can apply in the UK and Europe. As a result of altering the normal ranges for many blood tests, borderline and mild conditions can be excluded. There are many examples of such changes to normal ranges, those for **thyroid problems** being a particular example. A test that I frequently request is for free T4 (thyroxine), which, along with TSH (thyroid stimulating hormone), makes up a thyroid profile. Over my career I have requested and scrutinised probably thousands of thyroid profile results from both NHS and private laboratories. I am still surprised at the variety of normal ranges offered by different laboratories. The Doctors Laboratory to which I send blood samples, one of the largest private laboratories in Europe, advises a normal range for thyroxine of between 12 and 22 pmol/l (that is, 'pica moles' per litre). However, I have seen NHS normal ranges for the same test as low as 7 to 18 pmol/l. In parts of America the normal range for thyroxine is recommended to be between 15 and 30 pmol/l.

So, there can be enormous variations in what is a commonly requested test. In addition to the recommended normal ranges, there are many other factors that should be considered before deciding if a patient has an underactive or overactive thyroid gland. These include:

1. The human thyroid varies in weight from 8 to 50 grams – that is, a six-fold variation in size; this tends to add to confusion over the question, what is a patient's optimal function?

2. A patient's age can influence blood test results. Our thyroid activity reduces as we grow older. Yet in spite of this, the normal laboratory ranges are the same for all ages.

3. Those patients who are already taking thyroxine for hypothyroidism should have an adjusted normal range – that is, higher levels to allow for their thyroxine dosage. For this reason, many countries recommend two normal ranges. A common feature of thyroid results from American laboratories is to offer a normal range that is adjusted to the patients' age and thyroxine dosage. This unfortunately is not an approach seen in Europe.

4. When testing the T4 (thyroxine) of patients who are taking thyroxine, it is essential that they avoid their thyroxine for 24 hours prior to the test. This is recommended to avoid an artificially high result. A 10–15% increase can show in the T4 level if the patient tested is taking 100 micrograms or more on a daily basis. Unfortunately this is often not done in the UK.

Possibly, the only sure method of discovering a patient's normal range for thyroxine is to measure their thyroid hormone levels when they are symptom free. Unfortunately, this is not recommended as a routine, except with newborn babies. (Following birth, babies are tested to check for 'cretinism' – the absence of a thyroid gland.) A routine thyroid profile blood test for every citizen upon reaching adulthood at 18 years would be an invaluable, cost-cutting example of preventative medicine. A blood group test would be a useful addition, if not already known.

The four factors listed above, that can influence a diagnosis of an underactive thyroid, are only valid if the level of thyroxine (free T4) is measured. A popular and, I believe, incorrect view is that the free T4 test is only required when the level of TSH (thyroid stimulating hormone), which is a pituitary hormone, is abnormal. The TSH level by definition will rise when the thyroid is under-functioning. It is therefore seen as the most valuable test for thyroid function. A normal level is under 4.2 µg/l, but it can be in excess of 100 miu/l. However, as you will see below, there are occasions when this does not happen, and *both* hormone levels are low.

I see many patients who have never had a test for free T4 because their doctor or consultant is relying only on their TSH status for diagnosis and/ or monitoring the gland. This view seems to be unique to Europe; many Australian, Canadian and American test results emphasise the importance of free T4 and give it diagnostic priority over the TSH test. I have on many occasions treated patients with a free T4 as low as 5 pmol/l, yet with a 'normal' TSH. This low level of free T4 indicates hypothyroidism while the TSH level does not.

One explanation for this occurrence (low T4 and normal TSH) is the real possibility that the whole glandular or endocrine axis is depressed and the pituitary gland that secretes the TSH may also be under-functioning. Many practitioners believe that it is virtually impossible to have a single gland malfunctioning. When the thyroid is underactive, the adrenal glands are invariably likewise depressed. The ovaries are also frequently imbalanced; pre-menstrual syndrome is a very common symptom of hypothyroidism.

The protocol for thyroid testing in the UK is flawed and incomplete unless the free T4 test is included in the profile. It is my opinion that the TSH is diagnostically valid only with moderate to severe hypothyroidism. With mild or borderline thyroid problems, the TSH may not be an accurate or reliable guide for a diagnosis.

Unlike many health problems, the diagnosis and treatment of chronic fatigue are so controversial that I have seen patients who have suffered from their symptoms for over 20 years. In addition to any standard profile, there is a value in individual assessment using specialised test profiles. I will begin by describing the standard profile.

Standard test profile

My standard test profile is a non-specific and broad ranging test that looks at blood levels of the elements in the following list. Patients are requested to fast on water only, for 12 hours prior to the test.

Haematology

Haemoglobin
HCT (Haematocrit)
Red cell count
MCV (Mean corpuscular volume)
MCHC (Mean corpuscular haemoglobin concentration)
Platelet count
White cell count
Neutrophils
Lyphycytes
Monocytes
Eosinophils
Basophils
ESR (Erythrocyte sedimentation rate)
Vitamin B-12 (active)

Endocrinology

TSH (Thyroid stimulating hormone)
Free T4 (Thyroxine)
Free T3 (Triiodothyronine)

Biochemistry

Urea
Creatinine
Bilirubin
Alkaline phosphatase
Aspartatet transferase
Alamine transferase
LDH (Lactate dehydrogenase)
CK or CPK (Creatinine kinase)
Gamma GT or GGT (gamma glutamyl transpeptidase)
Total protein
Albumin
Globulin
Phosphate
Uric acid
Glucose
Triglycerides
Cholesterol
HDL cholesterol
LDL cholesterol
Iron
TIBC (Total iron binding capacity)
Transferin saturation
Ferritin

This profile consists of 40 tests which, as already outlined, can identify a wide range of disorders. However, many of the tests are designed to recognise or eliminate well-established health problems in terms of severity. Unfortunately, this means that early-stage, borderline conditions can sometimes be missed. Furthermore, as I have said earlier in the book, our blood chemistry tends to have priority status over many other organs and systems; levels in the organs are sacrificed to maintain healthy levels in the blood. This means that blood tests alone cannot tell us everything. Many cancers, for example, cannot be diagnosed with blood testing alone. I am sure that we all know of a friend or neighbour who died suddenly, the day after a routine, comprehensive health check had given him or her the 'all clear'.

Although there have been many attempts to define CFS over the last 50 years, it needs to be remembered that fatigue, like pain, is essentially a symptom. We have all experienced fatigue, whether resulting from overwork, insomnia, stress, infection or actual illness. We can all remember being tired. However, as with any symptoms, there are degrees of severity, ranging from being a little tired to completely exhausted up to a point of inertia. Chronic fatigue is a subjective symptom. It is by definition 'our' symptom and hence very difficult for another person to evaluate. A universally acceptable standard for fatigue with a scale of 1-10 would be very useful.

I believe that we have two methods of fairly accurately assessing our energy levels or fatigue severity. One is comparison with family, friends and fellow workers: you should be able to match their vitality fairly well; alarm bells can ring if you are always the first in a group to dream of bedtime. The second, and perhaps a more exact method of assessing available energy, is to remember how you used to feel, whether three or two months before or even years. Patients often recount examples of their fatigue, in terms of 'jobs they can no longer do', quite often within a small time frame of three to six months.

We can all remember an earlier life when, no matter how tired we became, we were normal and recovered after a good night's sleep. The type of disabling exhaustion suffered by many who have CFS is quite different from the transient tiredness that a good night's sleep or a holiday will resolve. In fact, very few patients with CFS feel alert and refreshed on rising. It is very often their worst time of day.

Chronic fatigue profile

Many practitioners request personalised blood test profiles from private laboratories. Such profiles offer a range of tests for diagnostic options. Specific groups of tests can provide specific information for areas of ill-health of special interest to the requesting practitioner. With my own 'chronic fatigue profile', the tests give results for most of the commonly seen causes of chronic fatigue (see chapter 3). Although these can be requested by GPs, I am often surprised at the number of patients I see who have never had such tests. My chronic fatigue profile consists of the following tests:

Haematology

- Haemoglobin
- HCT
- Red cell count
- MCV
- MCHC
- Platelet count
- White cell count
- Neutrophils
- Lyphocytes
- Monocytes
- Eosinophils
- Basophils
- ESR

Thyroid

- Free T4
- Free T3
- TSH

Biochemistry

- Glucose
- Uric acid
- Vitamin B-12 (active)
- Iron
- TIBC
- Ferritin

Although I send blood samples to various laboratories, I also frequently see test results that are provided by my patients' GPs. However, I very often need to request additional tests from private laboratories. As I have previously described, some tests are adequate for a diagnosis. However, all too often the results of previous tests fail to provide the necessary diagnostic clues to explain the type of exhaustion so commonly seen in CFS patients. As I have already explained, diagnosis is made easier when the tests' 'normal ranges' have been adjusted for the individual, taking into account factors such as age, sex, past health history, current stress-load and diet.

As you know if you are yourself a CFS sufferer, fatigue is never the only symptom. I believe that many of the exhausted sufferers of CFS in the UK are victims of multiple causes, this being one reason why CFS has for many years presented a diagnostic challenge. Although there have been many unsuccessful attempts by mainstream medicine over the last 50 years to identify a specific viral cause for CFS (or ME as it has been termed), the concept of several causes offers a more valid explanation for the great diversity of chronic fatigue syndrome symptoms.

Special testing

Given the premise that there can be multiple causes of CFS, just how can these be identified and measured?

Detailed case-history taking can reveal a great deal, in terms of the duration and severity of various symptoms. However, it can be very reassuring to an exhausted patient to have a test result confirm there is a treatable problem. This particularly applies if he/she has been prescribed anti-depressants and informed that the problem is 'all in the mind' or 'psychosomatic'. Apart from certain viral conditions and obscure neurological disorders, there are very few health problems that completely defy accurate medical diagnosis.

Patients frequently thank me for finding something wrong with them. CFS sufferers can begin to focus on recovery if they know the cause, or causes, of their symptoms. If a diagnosis is not available, such patients can believe themselves incurable. The concept of matching test results (blood, saliva, hair, urine) to a patient's symptoms, can offer a convincing and reassuring explanation for their problem.

Some patients express surprise that I should need to request diagnostic tests. They point out that I have written books on various topics and treated CFS for over 40 years. So why, they ask, are tests needed? The answer to such a question falls into six parts.

1. Although there are many hundreds of health problems with fatigue as a symptom, there are several commonly seen problems that can cause severe fatigue – anaemia, diabetes, hypoglycaemia, adrenal

exhaustion, and hypothyroidism. These need to be tested for at the outset, on the basis that they are the most likely and if you can identify the problem you can start to treat it. (Note, this list does not include the life-threatening diseases, which are not the subject of this book, but these do also have to be ruled out, of course, or suspicions raised and the patient referred to a specialist.) I do not favour guess work in diagnosis, particularly when confronted with an exhausted patient who has suffered for perhaps 10–20 years.

2. The diagnostic value of specific tests and groups of test can be understood. Fortunately with such tests, many health problems can be discounted when the results are normal, thus potentially saving time and money.

3. For my own guidance – a patient's test results can assist me in the areas of any appropriate nutritional advice, supplement choice and dosage requirements. There is no such person as a standard human being. All my patients have the annoying habit of being different in just about every area of health. This particularly applies to CFS which, as I have explained, can be a complex, multi-system condition.

4. Just as it is at times very useful and possible to equate a patient's test results with his/her symptoms, the initial test results can be a reliable basis for comparison with any subsequent results. This can serve to reassure the patient that real progress is being made, in spite of the occasional relapse.

5. I usually request blood tests every three months; in this way a recovery 'time-scale' can often be established based on progress to date.

6. Many people have suffered from chronic fatigue over so many years that they are unaware of just how they should feel when they are 'normal'. Test results when the patient is fully recovered will, however, provide a set of figures to match their progress and that they can rely on for any future test comparisons. Our blood chemistry can provide reassuring statistics to confirm that all is well and normal. This assumes that a patient's final test results and symptoms match his/her own definition of 'normal'.

This section began with the question, 'So why are tests needed?' In addition to the general points that I have listed, it will become very obvious why the appropriate selection of special tests is an essential component of CFS diagnosis and treatment when you look through the tests described below.

Why are many special tests not available with the NHS?

We are encouraged to believe that modern hospital testing and treatment, whether with the use of drugs or surgery, offers state of the art, comprehensive care. Yet readers may be surprised to learn that there are many tests and treatments that are not available under mainstream medicine. Many of the tests that I request to assist the diagnosis and treatment of chronic fatigue are only available from specialised private laboratories.

Certain blood tests are classed as 'special request' tests by the NHS. Unfortunately, their selection is not always based on patient or clinical considerations. Their choice is usually determined by commercial priority. In simple language, the tests cost too much for general use.

There are other cost considerations. Within the NHS, certain prescriptions are termed 'free prescriptions'. These are given to those people who have a lifelong need for a particular treatment (for example, for Parkinsonism, diabetes or hypothyroidism). Patients get not only their levodopa, insulin, thyroxine etc, free but all their other prescriptions too. This can be an expensive business. Unfortunately, one of the results of ongoing cost-cutting is the lowering of the normal ranges for hypothyroidism tests (the UK's are now probably the lowest in the world) and consequently, the under-diagnosis and treatment of hypothyroidism.

I usually refer my patients' tests to the Doctors Laboratory in Wimpole Street. Their normal range for free T4 is 12 to 22 pmol/l. I have seen patients' results from many parts of Britain, and different area health authorities; the lowest normal range I have seen was 7.5–18.00 pmol/l, but the range is frequently 8 or 9 to 20 pmol/l. To put these figures into context, the average free T4 for all ages is 16.9 pmol/l. These recommended ranges do not allow much scope for diagnosing borderline or sub-thyroid patients. It has been estimated that there may be up to 500,000 people in the UK who are suffering the effects of an under-functioning thyroid gland, the chief symptom of which is fatigue.

When assessing thyroid function, the patient's age becomes relevant. Our thyroid output reduces as we age. It is therefore quite possible for a 70-year-old with a T4 level of 9 pmol/l to feel well. However, a 20-year-old with the same level would probably be exhausted.

NHS testing

Many of my patients have supportive and co-operative GPs who are willing to request blood tests for their patients and allow me to see the results. I prefer to work with GPs whenever possible because:

1. I request, and usually obtain, access to all a patient's past test results. Even when the results are labelled NAD (no abnormality detected), they can provide a useful basis for comparison with the latest tests, always remembering that the NHS view of 'normal' tends to differ from my view.

2. I am very rarely consulted by CFS patients who are not taking prescription drugs. Such drugs can include anti-depressants, anti-cholesterol drugs (statins), beta-blockers (prescribed for anxiety, high blood pressure, migraine, angina, palpitations and hyperthyroidism), analgesics (pain killers), sleeping tablets and hormone replacement therapy. It can be very helpful to liaise with a patient's GP before I decide to offer alternatives to prescription drugs or to prescribe supplements that may compromise the efficiency of the drugs. However, it needs to be remembered that the majority of drugs are only prescribed for symptom relief.

3. As I have stated elsewhere, I do not regard naturopaths like myself as replacement GPs. Nor do I provide a naturopathic A & E service for my patients. Acute and emergency conditions are usually treated effectively by mainstream medicine within the NHS. I prefer to work with GPs, as such co-operation can be reassuring to an already stressed and exhausted patient. To present CFS patients with an 'either/or' situation when choosing a practitioner or therapy is neither appropriate nor advisable. I have always preferred the term

'complementary medicine' to 'alternative medicine'. It is perhaps worth remembering that complementary can be defined as meaning supportive, harmonious and reciprocal. It is unfortunate that the word complementary is so often confused with complimentary.

4. The problem of drug side-effects with CFS patients is an area that I need at times to discuss with patients and their GPs. Many drugs have fatigue listed as a major side-effect. Unfortunately, when patients are taking a 'cocktail' of several drugs, the total combined side-effects from such a mix are virtually unknown, and simply not researched or disclosed by the drug manufacturers. When patients are taking several different drugs for symptom relief, vital diagnostic clues can easily be missed or misinterpreted.

5. I have found that a patient's drugs can often be reduced or discontinued, with his/her GP's support. Then a more precise indication of his/her response to my treatment, particularly when involving replacement supplements, can become apparent.

SPECIAL TESTS DESCRIBED

This section includes tests that various laboratories provide to look into the cause or causes of CFS, as outlined in chapters 3 and 4. If this can be achieved, then a systematic and ultimately effective treatment strategy can be devised, with a good chance of success.

Active vitamin B-12
Ferritin
Red cell minerals
Omega-3/Omega-6
ATP profile (CFS profile)
Female hormone profile
Adrenal stress profile

Allergy testing
Gut fermentation profile
Gut permeability – using
    PEG400
Glucose tolerance test
Glucometre use

Active vitamin B-12

Vitamin B-12 deficiency is usually linked to pernicious anaemia. Some people consider that pernicious anaemia is a general description for vitamin

B-12 deficiency, but there are many people who suffer from the symptoms of B-12 deficiency, yet do not have pernicious anaemia. 'Pernicious' means harmful, dangerous or lethal. 'Pernicious anaemia' is defined as being harmful anaemia 'caused by impaired intestinal absorption of vitamin B-12 due to lack of availability of intrinsic factor' (*Dorland's Illustrated Medical Dictionary* 1994). Intrinsic factor is a protein that is released by special cells in the stomach lining and combines with B-12 in food, with the aid of pancreatic proteases in the small intestine; this B-12 intrinsic-factor complex travels to the ileum (the last section of the small intestine), where cells absorb it into the blood stream. Any absorbed vitamin B-12 that is not needed immediately is stored in the liver. The process is summarised here in Figure 5.1.

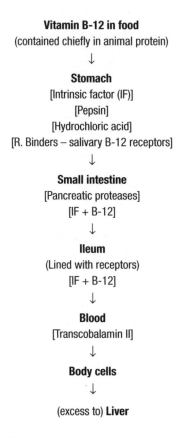

Vitamin B-12 in food
(contained chiefly in animal protein)
↓

Stomach
[Intrinsic factor (IF)]
[Pepsin]
[Hydrochloric acid]
[R. Binders – salivary B-12 receptors]
↓

Small intestine
[Pancreatic proteases]
[IF + B-12]
↓

Ileum
(Lined with receptors)
[IF + B-12]
↓

Blood
[Transcobalamin II]
↓

Body cells
↓

(excess to) **Liver**

Figure 5.1: Vitamin B-12 metabolism

A high percentage of people with vitamin B-12 deficiency eat sufficient amounts of the vitamin. Their problem is that, for various reasons, their body cannot absorb or make use of it. This may be owing to lack of intrinsic factor, but a problem at any stage in the process shown in Figure 5.1 (page 113) can reduce absorption. Other causes include:

Reduced stomach acid (atrophic gastritis) – This involves inflammation of the stomach lining and a reduced ability to separate vitamin B-12 from food protein. Ant-acids and other medications are known to contribute to this deficiency.

Stomach surgery – This may be for weight loss (gastric bypass) or complete or partial stomach removal for tumours etc. The total number of cells that release the essential hydrochloric acid and intrinsic factor is consequently reduced.

Gastro-intestinal inflammation – This can be due to Crohn's disease, coeliac disease (gluten intolerance), alcohol, drugs for stomach ulcer, drugs for diabetes, and various toxins including mercury and nitrous oxide exposure (laughing gas).

Unfortunately, taking oral supplements of vitamin B-12 is no guarantee of normal absorption. The American National Institute of Health has stated that only 10 micrograms of a 500 microgram supplement are in fact absorbed by a healthy person – that is, someone who does not have problems with intrinsic factor or stomach atrophy. For this reason vitamin B-12 injections often need to be prescribed.

Active vitamin B-12 is a relatively new test, which needs to be differentiated from the longstanding, standard test for vitamin B-12 used in the NHS, which looks at 'total B-12' – that is, *all* the vitamin B-12 in a patient's blood. The principle behind the new test is that not all B-12 is able to travel into the cells for DNA synthesis; only the 10–30% known as 'halotranscobalamin' or 'active B-12' can be so used. It therefore makes sense to measure just the proportion of B-12 that will contribute to our health.

Before the active B-12 test became available, the urinary MMA (methylmalonic acid) was used, but only rarely in the NHS. Raised levels of this acid are present with a deficiency of vitamin B-12.

One other test can indicate vitamin B-12 deficiency. A raised level of homocysteine (using the Hcy test) in the blood can point to vitamin B-12 deficiency. Unfortunately, it is also elevated with low levels of vitamin B-6 and folic acid.

On a final point, American researchers, utilising a breath test to identify B-12 deficiency, have concluded that 40% of Americans are suffering from vitamin B12 deficiency.

Tests for iron-deficient anaemia

Iron-deficient anaemia (IDA) is by far the commonest type of anaemia (see chapter 3, page 41). Unfortunately, as I have outlined below, the medical diagnosis and subsequent treatment of IDA are flawed and questionable. A view that is frequently expressed is that GPs can quite easily diagnose and treat IDA, with standard blood tests (haemoglobin and iron) and by prescribing iron preparations (eg ferrous sulphate). I hope it be clear from the section that follows that the ferritin test is the best indicator for iron status.

I often see very fatigued patients with chronic IDA, who have been reassured, often repeatedly over several years, that their blood tests are normal. Not surprisingly, such patients are depressed as well as exhausted. A prescription for anti-depressants is frequently their sole treatment option. How can this happen to many thousands of chronically fatigued people? I have yet to see a depressed person who was full of energy. The fatigue usually precedes the depression, which often lifts as energy improves.

As I have already described, the diagnostic protocol of many overworked GPs is to base their diagnosis entirely on blood test findings and to thereby avoid, if possible, time-consuming discussions over symptoms, with their patients. This all too frequently applies to the diagnosis of IDA. Diagnosis solely from blood test results *could* work well if the two requirements I mentioned earlier in the chapter are met:

1. The test selection is matched with the patient's symptoms and health history.
2. Interpretation of the test results takes into account the variety and severity of the patient's symptoms.

The symptoms of IDA can include hair loss, pallor, headaches, depression, fatigue, breathlessness, palpitations, poor immunity, low body temperature, reduced thyroid output, reduced libido, bruising, poor concentration, and learning difficulties in children.

The standard NHS profile for investigating possible IDA is usually full blood count (FBC), plus (but not always) haemoglobin and serum iron levels. Unfortunately such tests do not fulfil the two requirements stated; they are insufficient and the interpretation is therefore of little value for an accurate diagnosis. Furthermore, several factors serve to compromise the reliability of these three tests. These include the female menstrual cycle, the presence of an infection or stress when taking the blood sample, and the time of day the blood is taken. Iron in the blood can vary by as much as 30% throughout 24 hours. The level is higher in the morning and lower in the evening. NHS testing is standard, and does not take variations within and between people into account.

The most accurate test to identify a patient's iron status is bone marrow aspiration and biopsy. However, this is an invasive procedure and the discomfort to the patient, the high cost of the test and the real risk of infection, serve to make this a very rarely requested test. Assuming it to be 100% accurate in detecting IDA, other tests rate as follows:

ferritin – 90% accuracy
serum iron + haemoglobin – 41% accuracy

Ferritin is an iron-containing protein. Around 30% of our available iron is stored as ferritin with the remaining 70% being present in the haemoglobin in our red blood cells. Given its accuracy, it is puzzling that ferritin testing – which is highly regarded by many practitioners and biochemists and is readily available – is so infrequently requested by GPs. Possible reasons include:

1. Very few GPs are familiar with ferritin testing and its special value when diagnosing IDA, having been trained to accept that the haemoglobin, FBC and serum iron profile is adequate and reliable.
2. Many health authorities within the NHS have become very cash-flow conscious and the ferritin test is often defined as a 'special request test', as a result of its cost.

3. Ferritin tests are regarded as expensive; this is because of the high cost of the actual ferritin test kit. Private laboratories may charge £50 plus phlebotomy for a single ferritin test, yet offer full biochemistry plus haematology profiles consisting of 40+ tests for around £60.

4. I have heard GPs complain that they have requested the ferritin test, only to be informed by the laboratory staff that they are not permitted to test for ferritin when a patient's haemoglobin is normal.

Normal ranges for the ferritin test

Even when a patient's ferritin has been tested, problems arise over how to interpret the results. When *is* blood ferritin too low? The standard normal reference range advised for ferritin by the NHS laboratories is between 12 and 150 µg/l (micrograms per litre). Many private laboratories advise a range of between 28 and 250 µg/l. Practitioners who regularly request, and diagnose from, ferritin results prefer a level over 40 µg/l before excluding IDA. In men, the level of ferritin in blood serum increases with age, and in patients of both sexes over 65 years a level under 45 µg/l can indicate IDA.

There is another, often overlooked, factor that makes the ferritin test better for diagnosis than the standard tests for IDA: to keep our blood healthy, our body initially uses iron stored in tissue (ferritin) when we are not taking in enough iron, or losing iron due to blood loss. This can apply particularly in the early stages of IDA, when the typical symptoms are present, yet the haemoglobin and iron levels in the blood can still be within the normal ranges. This characteristic has been termed 'tissue anaemia' – that is, low reserves with normal blood levels.

As I have mentioned before, blood takes precedence over body tissues and organs when a nutrient is in short supply. This can apply, in particular, to minerals. For example, someone with osteoporosis may have a normal level of calcium in the blood but a deficient level in the bones. This is why ferritin levels in the tissues may not match those in the blood in IDA.

For diagnosis, the generally held view is that symptoms of IDA only appear when the haemoglobin level falls below 10 g/dl (the standard units for measuring iron). I believe this to be incorrect. I have seen many chronically fatigued patients with normal haemoglobins and serum irons, but with low blood ferritin. The symptoms of these patients invariably improve following treatment for IDA, but it may need up to six months of treatment.

The anaemias of chronic diseases (ACD)

The anaemias of chronic disease tend to occur with malignancies, infections and inflammatory disorders, and are therefore outside the scope of this book. In their case, ferritin testing would not be a diagnostic priority. ACDs also include other anaemias (including pernicious anaemia), which I have covered elsewhere. It is generally accepted by laboratory workers and doctors that when iron-deficiency anaemias (IDA) is diagnosed, to prescribe treatment without identifying the cause or causes constitutes gross negligence. IDA is generally caused by blood loss (see chapter 3, page 41), and if there is no obvious blood loss (such as excessively heavy periods), this must be investigated. If I suspect cancer, I refer that patient to his/her GP with a report.

I have discussed our role as naturopaths, when diagnosing and treating IDA, with many colleagues. The view frequently expressed is that GPs can quite easily diagnose the presence of IDA with standard blood tests (haemoglobin and iron). They can also prescribe a variety of iron preparations (such as ferrous sulphate) to top-up the haemoglobin. It therefore only remains for naturopaths to contribute to the patient's treatment with nutritional advice (iron-rich foods etc) and synergistic nutritional support if needed. As I have explained earlier in the book, my experience is that IDA is often *not* diagnosed by GPs.

Red cell mineral testing

Red cell mineral testing is seen as the preferred test for assessing a patient's mineral status. The profile includes the following minerals:

Red cell potassium	Red cell zinc
Red cell magnesium	Red cell copper
Red cell calcium	Red cell selenium
Red cell manganese	Red cell chromium

Essential red cell fatty acids – omega-3 to omega-6 ratio

This very useful test is provided by the Doctors Laboratory in Wimpole Street, central London. To quote (for a second time) from their latest laboratory guide:

> *Omega-3 is the name given to a family of polyunsaturated fatty acids, which the body needs but cannot manufacture itself. Omega-3 fats are used as the building blocks for fat-derived hormones such as prostaglandins and leukotrienes. The hormones with an omega-3 base tend to reduce inflammation, while those that have an omega-6 base increase inflammation. In the cell membrane the competition between these two essential fats has a direct bearing on the type of local hormone produced and the level of inflammation in the cell.*

> *The omega-6 to omega-3 ratio in the cell membranes is key to the development of inflammatory disorders such as rheumatoid arthritis and heart disease. Diets low in oily fish and high in grains will promote inflammation and affect good health. The ratio of omega-6 to omega-3 in the West is around 15 to 1, fifteen times more omega-6 on the cell membrane promoting inflammation. Having twice as much omega-6 is considered by most experts to be the optimal amount but a ratio of 2:1 is not easy to produce by diet alone. Many people are aware of the health benefits of omega-3 but the supplementation to achieve optimal health is erratic. Being able to test for essential red cell fatty acids (omega-6/omega-3 ratio) identifies a person's current status and is sufficiently specific to allow an accurate supplementation recommendation to be made.*

> *Results show the omega ratio with a clear recommendation for the required level of omega supplementation (if any) to achieve optimal levels.*

CFS profile for mitochondrial failure

The CFS profile for mitochondrial failure is a group of four tests designed by Dr John McLaren-Howard at the Acumen laboratory in Devon. It is seen by many as the definitive test for identifying the reasons for CFS.

As described in chapter 3 (see page 40), the universal currency of our energy is known as ATP (adenosine triphosphate). The ATP is supplied by the mitochondria within every cell in our bodies; the functioning of the mitochondria is reflected in the test.

There is growing support for the idea that CFS results from mitochondrial failure. To understand what this might be and why testing for it is important, we need to know more about what the mitochondria are. There are up to 3000 in each of our cells. They are the ultimate energy producers within the cells, and they also distribute our energy.

The process whereby energy is abstracted from our food, ultimately generating ATP, is known as the 'electron transport chain'; it is yet to be fully understood. The mitochondria use oxygen as an oxidising agent to produce energy. Unfortunately, around 1% of the oxygen we breathe is converted into corrosive oxygen materials, such as superoxide and hydrogen peroxide. The mitochondria have an effective anti-oxidation system, made up of antioxidants. These include superoxide dismutase, glutathione peroxidise, lipoic acid, co-enzyme Q-10 and L-carnitine. (Still with me?) Together they protect the mitochondria against oxidative stress and injury.

To understand the detail and importance of these processes I must refer you to Dr Sarah Myhill's book (see Further reading), but I have included two typical sets of results here (see Figures 5.2 (pages 122–3) and 5.3 (pages 124–5)) which serve to explain many of the issues. Patient number 1 is symptom-free; patient number 2 has CFS. The 'comments' on these sample results highlight the differences between normal and abnormal levels.

I will conclude with a quotation from Dr Myhill. She states that, 'The joy of the ATP profiles test is that we now have an objective test for chronic fatigue syndrome, which clearly shows this illness has a physical basis.'

Female hormone profile (saliva)

This endocrine profile – supplied by Genova Diagnostics – comprises 12 saliva samples over the course of one menstrual cycle. It is recommended for pre-menopausal women. The following are analysed:

Progesterone   Testosterone
Oestradiol   Progesterone/Oestradiol ratio

Saliva testing of these three hormones, unlike blood testing, measures the free un-bound fraction of each hormone. Imbalances in the three hormones can produce a range of symptoms, CFS being one of these.

Adrenal stress profile (saliva)

I request this saliva test on a regular basis for my CFS patients. It involves measuring cortisol and DHEA (dehydroepiandrosterone) (see pages 52–54) in four samples throughout one day. It gives a valuable indication of stress handling status and adrenal fatigue, which are common features of chronic fatigue and stress.

The measuring of the adrenal hormones cortisol and DHEA in the saliva has been the subject of many research projects in recent years, with particular reference to comparisons with testing these hormones in the blood, and the significance of the 'cortisol awakening response', or CAR, which is a profound increase in cortisol on waking, possible caused by blood sugar changes.

The *Journal of Clinical Endocrinal Metabolism* reported in October 2009: 'The measurement of cortisol in saliva is a simple, reproducible and reliable test to evaluate the normal and disordered control of the hypothalamic-pituitary-adrenal (HPA) axis. There are a variety of simple methods to obtain saliva samples without stress, making this a robust test applicable to many different experimental and clinical situations.'

The *British Journal of Psychiatry* carried an article in February 2004 entitled 'Salivary cortisol response to awakening in chronic fatigue syndrome' which said: 'There is accumulating evidence of HPA axis disturbance in CFS. The salivary cortisol response to awakening has been described recently as a non-invasive test of the capacity of the HPA axis to respond to stress.'

Allergy testing

To demonstrate the complexity and diversity involved in allergy testing, I have included profile lists of the blood tests available from the Doctors

ATP (adenosine triphosphate), studies on neutrophils

ATP is hydrolysed to ADP and phosphate as the major energy source in muscle and other tissues. It is regenerated by oxidative phosphorylation of ADP in the mitochondria. When aerobic metabolism provides insufficient energy, extra ATP is generated during the anaerobic breakdown of glucose to lactic acid. ATP reactions require magnesium. ADP to ATP conversion can be blocked by environmental contaminants as can the translocator [TL] in the mitochondrial membrane. [TL] efficiency is also sensitive to pH and other metabolic-factor changes. [TL] defects may demand excessive ADP to AMP conversion (not re-converted to ADP or through to ATP). Defects in Mg-ATP, ADP – ATP conversion and enryme or [TL] blocking can all result in **chronic fatigue – a factor in any disease where biochemical energy availability is reduced.**

ATP whole cells:

With excess Mg added	**1.92** nmol/10^6 cells	1.6–2.9
(Standard method of measuring ATP)		
Endogenous Mg only	**1.15** nmol/10^6 cells	0.9–2.7
(Measured ATP result is lowered during intracellular magnesium deficiency)		
Ratio ATP/ATP^{Mg}	**0.6**	>0.65

ADP to ATP conversion efficiency (whole cells):

ATP^{Mg} (from above)	**1.92** nmol/10^6 cells	(1*)	1.6–2.9
ATP^{Mg} (inhibitor present)	**0.08** nmol/10^6 cells	(2*)	<0.3
ATP^{Mg} (inhibitor removed)	**1.37** nmol/10^6 cells	(3*)	>1.4
ADP to ATP efficiency [(3* − 2*0/(1* − 2*)] x 100 = **70.1%**		**>60**	
Blocking of active sites (2*/1*) x 100 = **4.2%**		**up to 14**	

ADP-ATP TRANSLOCATOR [TL] (mitochondria, not whole cells):

	ATP (pmol/10^6 cells)	**Ref. range**	**change %**	**ref. range**
Start	**366**	290–700		
[TL] 'out'	**552**	410–950	**50.8**	over 35% (*Increase*)
				(in-vitro test) reflects ATP supply for cytoplasm
[TL] 'in'	**140**	140–330	**58.3**	55 to 75% (*Decrease*)
				(in-vitro test) reflects normal use of ATP on energy demand

---

Comments Rather low ATP-related magnesium: Otherwise-normal ATP profile.

Figure 5.2a: Typical mitochondrial function profile of a healthy individual

Chapter 5

<u>Superoxide Dismutase Studies</u>

A functional test looks at the in-vitro efficiency of the patient's red cell superoxide dismutase (SOD) when their neutrophil superoxide production is maximally stimulated. The activity of the individual forms of SOD are explored. General cell protection from damage by superoxide is provided by intracellular zinc:copper-SOD (Zn/Cu-SOD). Mitochondria are protected by manganese-dependent SOD (Mn-SOD). Extracellular SOD (EC-SOD – another Zn/Cu SODase) protects the nitric oxide pathways that relax vascular smooth muscle.

For each form of SODase, genetic variations are known, mutations can occur during excessive oxidative stress on DNA and polymorphisms can occur. DNA adducts can chemically block these genes.

Blood test results:

Test	Result	Units	Reference range
Functional test	38	%	Over 40 (mostly 41–47)
Zn/Cu-SOD	216	Enzyme activity (u)	240–410
Mn-SOD	142	Enzyme activity (u)	125–208
EC-SOD	44	Enzyme activity (u)	28–70

Gene studies:

SOD form	Gene(s)	Comments
Zn/Cu-SOD Coded on chromosome 21	Mild blocking (see DNA-adducts)	Low enzyme activity
Mn-SOD Coded on chromosome 6	Normal	Normal enzyme activity
EC-SOD Coded on chromosome 4	Normal	Normal enzyme activity

Figure 5.2b: Typical mitochondrial function profile of a healthy individual (cont'd)

ATP (adenosine triphosphate), studies on neutrophils

ATP is hydrolysed to ADP and phosphate as the major energy source in muscle and other tissues. It is regenerated by oxidative phosphorylation of ADP in the mitochondria. When aerobic metabolism provides insufficient energy, extra ATP is generated during the anaerobic breakdown of glucose to lactic acid. ATP reactions require magnesium. ADP to ATP conversion can be blocked by environmental contaminants as can the translocator [TL] in the mitochondrial membrane. [TL] efficiency is also sensitive to pH and other metabolic-factor changes. [TL] defects may demand excessive ADP to AMP conversion (not re-converted to ADP or through to ATP). Defects in Mg-ATP, ADP – ATP conversion and enryme or [TL] blocking can all result in **chronic fatigue – a factor in any disease where biochemical energy availability is reduced.**

ATP whole cells:

With excess Mg added	**1.28** nmol/10^6 cells	1.6–2.9
(Standard method of measuring ATP)		
Endogenous Mg only	**0.65** nmol/10^6 cells	0.9–2.7
(Measured ATP result is lowered during intracellular magnesium deficiency)		
Ratio ATP/ATP^{Mg}	**0.51**	>0.65

ADP to ATP conversion efficiency (whole cells):

ATP^{Mg} (from above)	**1.28** nmol/10^6 cells	(1*)	1.6–2.9
ATP^{Mg} (inhibitor present)	**0.08** nmol/10^6 cells	(2*)	<0.3
ATP^{Mg} (inhibitor removed)	**0.58** nmol/10^6 cells	(3*)	>1.4

ADP to ATP efficiency $[(3^* - 2^*0/(1^* - 2^*)] \times 100 = $ **41.7%**   **>60**

Blocking of active sites $(2^*/1^*) \times 100 = $ **6.3%**   **up to 14**

ADP-ATP TRANSLOCATOR [TL] (mitochondria, not whole cells):

	ATP (pmol/10^6 cells)	**Ref. range**	**change %**	**ref. range**
Start	**215**	290–700		
[TL] '*out*'	**262**	410–950	**21.9**	over 35% (*Increase*)
				(in-vitro test) reflects ATP supply for cytoplasm
[TL] '*in*'	**45**	140–330	**79.1**	55 to 75% (*Decrease*)
				(in-vitro test) reflects normal use of ATP on energy demand

---

Comments	Very low whole-cell ATP	Low ATP-related magnesium
	No significant blocking of active sites	Very poor ADP to ATP re-conversion
	Very low mt-ATP and very poor provision of ATP	
	Rapid depletion of ATP on increased energy demand.	

Figure 5.3a: Typical mitochondrial function profile of a patient with CFS

<u>Superoxide Dismutase Studies</u>

A functional test looks at the in-vitro efficiency of the patient's red cell superoxide dismutase (SOD) when their neutrophil superoxide production is maximally stimulated. The activity of the individual forms of SOD are explored. General cell protection from damage by superoxide is provided by intracellular zinc:copper-SOD (Zn/Cu-SOD). Mitochondria are protected by manganese-dependent SOD (Mn-SOD). Extracellular SOD (EC-SOD – another Zn/Cu SODase) protects the nitric oxide pathways that relax vascular smooth muscle.

For each form of SODase, genetic variations are known, mutations can occur during excessive oxidative stress on DNA and polymorphisms can occur. DNA adducts can chemically block these genes.

Blood test results:

Test	Result	Units	Reference range
Functional test	36	%	Over 40 (mostly 41–47)
Zn/Cu-SOD	210	Enzyme activity (u)	240–410
Mn-SOD	132	Enzyme activity (u)	125–208
EC-SOD	24	Enzyme activity (u)	28–70

Gene studies:

SOD form	Gene(s)	Comments
Zn/Cu-SOD Coded on chromosome 21	Normal	Low enzyme activity
Mn-SOD Coded on chromosome 6	Normal	Normal enzyme activity
EC-SOD Coded on chromosome 4	Normal	Normal enzyme activity

Figure 5.3b: Typical mitochondrial function profile of a patient with CFS (cont'd)

Laboratory in London. They provide a total of 19 different profiles (groups of tests), ranging in price from £96 to £400. Testing for individual allergens can also be requested as follows:

Individual foods (32 tests)
Grass pollens (25 tests)
Weed pollens (36 tests)
Tree pollens (157 tests)
Milk and milk proteins (14 tests)
Micro-organisms (35 tests)
Epidermal and animal protein (52 tests)
Insects (12 tests)
Venoms (8 tests)
Drugs (14 tests)
Occupational (22 tests)
Parasites (3 tests).

Allergy testing improves continuously and it can provide useful clues to explain many symptoms. Useful profiles include:

Eczema-provoking allergens profile
Food and inhalants profile
Children's panel profile
Inhalants alone profile
Antibiotics profile
Rhinitis-provoking profile.

Unless an allergy is a lifelong problem – such as gluten or lactose intolerance – a diagnostic approach that attempts to identify a patient's immune efficiency and the cause of their allergy can be more rewarding than reliance on extensive allergy testing. This could involve testing for candidiasis, leaky gut, digestive enzymes and toxic load.

Environmental toxins

Xenobiotics is a word that describes any chemicals or molecules that are foreign to our metabolism.

Chapter 5

'Total load' is the concept that the sum of factors that can adversely influence our metabolism all need to be taken into account. W J Rea, in *Chemical Sensitivity, Volume 4* has outlined the contributors to this phenomenon as follows:

Xenobiotics (insecticides, herbicides, drugs, solvents, metals etc)
Infections (streptococcus, parasites etc)
Toxins (ergot (a fungus), heavy metals etc)
Biological inhalants (moulds, algae, pollens etc)
Physical phenomena (electromagnetic fields etc)
Lifestyle (alcohol, tobacco, recreational drugs etc)
Mechanical problems (nasal, intestinal etc)
Hormonal imbalances (DHEA, cortisol, oestrogen etc)
Psycho-social factors (stress, belief systems etc).

Rea's findings from over 20,000 patients with chemical sensitivity, pointed to nutritional abnormalities being common amongst them. He confirmed that nutritional intervention, nutrient supplementation and total load awareness needed to be part of any treatment programme. A person's exposure to toxins is an important element in this. When taking a CFS sufferer's history, it is therefore vital to include exposure to poisons over time. Make sure your practitioner is aware of any toxins you may have been exposed to.

As described in chapter 4, many toxins can contribute to CFS. These can be tested for and identified in our environment. It can be of value to assess an individual's toxic load. The following factors may need to be covered:

Environmental – Air quality, noise, low-frequency sound (page 75) etc
Home – Heating and ventilation, paints, pesticides, cleaning chemicals, carpets, allergens, moulds, water quality etc
Personal – Tobacco, alcohol, recreational drugs, stress handling, exercise etc
Occupational – Work stresses, air quality, toxic chemicals etc
Diet – Junk foods, general food quality, protein content, allergies etc
Medicines – Prescription and over the counter
Dental work - Mercury amalgams
Childhood influences – Passive smoking, mother's health etc.

Intestinal health

There are approximately 400 species of micro-organisms present in the human intestine. This population constitutes one of largest systems in the body, with a total weight of around 6 pounds (that is, around 2.75 kilograms). This vast collection of beneficial microbes is involved in our metabolic maintenance and synthesis of vitamins (including biotin, many of the B vitamins, vitamin K, and para-aminobenzoic acid, or 'PABA'). They reduce toxins, support immune efficiency and produce short-chain fatty acids (SCFAs) (see Glossary) from fibre.

However, antibiotics and other influences may upset the balance of these microbes and lead to the overgrowth of some at the expense of others. This relates in particular to the candidas – yeasts that can also take a fungal form and penetrate the lining of the gut, causing what is known as a 'leaky gut' (see page 62).

The gut fermentation profile

This is the group of tests used to investigate possible fermentation in the small intestine. It includes a definitive diagnosis for *Candida albicans*. If there is an overgrowth of yeast cells (candida etc) in the gut, these will cause any glucose the patient has eaten to ferment, thereby converting glucose to alcohol (ethanol), which then passes into the blood stream. The test therefore involves the patient swallowing a certain amount of glucose on an empty stomach and then testing his/her blood after an hour to see if it contains alcohol. To ensure that at least some of the glucose passes into the patient's duodenum, a proportion of the glucose taken is encased in hardened gelatine capsules.

Procedure

The patient avoids alcohol for at least 24 hours prior to the test and needs to fast completely for at least three hours before it begins. Early in the day he/she attends the surgery and is given 1 gram of glucose contained in two capsules (2×500 milligram capsules) together with 4 grams of glucose dissolved in 80–100 millilitres of water (that is, 5% glucose solution). A small (2 millilitres) blood sample is taken after 60 minutes. The blood is then sent to a laboratory to test the level of ethanol (Biolab in central London does this). Any ethanol present confirms the presence of yeast (candidiasis) and bacterial 'dysbiosis', or imbalance. The test results also include short-chain fatty acids and related substances (SCFAs), which can be absorbed and used for energy; they also help to maintain intestinal health.

Probiotics and prebiotics

'Probiotic' means 'for life', and is used to describe the beneficial microbes that serve to improve the intestinal microbial balance and provide immune system support, examples being lactobacilli and bifido bacteria. 'Prebiotics' are the foods that the probiotics live on. They consist chiefly of plant material (fermentable starches) that occurs particularly in asparagus, artichoke, chicory, onion, bananas and soya. Both prebiotics and probiotics are prescribed in combination for a wide range of gastro-intestinal conditions. Not surprisingly these beneficial bacteria can be supportive when treating chronic fatigue symptoms.

Gut permeability test – Peg test or 'leaky gut' test

The gut permeability test is based on the concept that a 'leaky gut' will allow molecules of foods that are larger than could normally be absorbed to pass into the blood stream. It requires the patient to take a small drink at home, containing polyethylene glycol (PEG), a substance which cannot be absorbed, but passes out directly to the patient's bladder. Added to the PEG are 11 substances that have different sized molecules; the normal recovery range is known for each molecule. The patient is required to measure the amount of urine passed over the six hours following the drink. A small sample of the urine taken at the end of the six-hour period, in addition to a figure for the total amount passed, is sent to the laboratory. (Again, Biolab do this analysis.)

This elegant and very simple test, which the patient does at home, serves to identify a leaky gut or, the opposite, malabsorption. I have chosen three profiles (Figure 5.4) that are typical of patients with the following diagnoses: A – Leaky gut ; B – Malabsorption; and C – Normal gut to illustrate test findings.

Mannitol-lactulose test

This is another test for intestinal permeability. It uses a standard amount of a mixture of two sugars – lactulose and mannitol. In a healthy person, only a

A: Leaky Gut   Recovery in urine (6 hour collection)

Fraction	Molecular weight	Dose (Mg)	Mg	%	Reference range
1	198	4.0	1.4	**35.9**	26.6–33.4
2	242	9.0	3.2	**35.7**	26.5–31.6
3	286	39.0	13.3	**34.1**	25.2–29.4
4	330	96.0	28.2	**29.4**	21.1–25.0
5	374	157.0	41.6	**26.5**	17.9–22.0
6	418	171.0	32.7	**19.1**	12.5–16.2
7	462	176.0	22.2	**12.6**	6.4–10.8
8	506	145.0	14.1	**9.7**	3.6–6.0
9	550	105.0	6.3	**6.0**	1.0–2.4
10	594	67.0	1.6	**2.4**	Up to 1.4
11	638	31.0	0.4	**1.2**	Up to 0.7
	TOTAL:	**1000.0**	**165.0**	**16.5**	**10.0–13.3%**

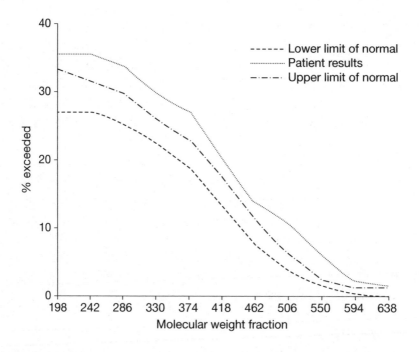

Figure 5.4a: Typical profile for leaky gut

B: Malabsorption   Recovery in urine (6 hour collection)

Fraction	Molecular weight	Dose (Mg)	Mg	%	Reference range
1	198	4.0	1.0	**24.9**	26.6–33.4
2	242	9.0	2.2	**24.1**	26.5–31.6
3	286	39.0	9.0	**23.2**	25.2–29.4
4	330	96.0	15.4	**16.0**	21.1–25.0
5	374	157.0	14.8	**9.4**	17.9–22.0
6	418	171.0	8.2	**4.8**	12.5–16.2
7	462	176.0	3.9	**2.2**	6.4–10.8
8	506	145.0	1.5	**1.0**	3.6–6.0
9	550	105.0	0.4	**0.4**	1.0–2.4
10	594	67.0	0.0	**0.0**	Up to 1.4
11	638	31.0	0.0	**0.0**	Up to 0.7
	TOTAL:	**1000.0**	**56.3**	**5.6**	**10.0–13.3%**

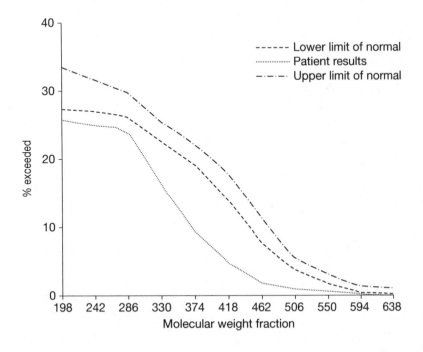

Figure 5.4b: Typical profile for malabsorption

C: Normal   Recovery in urine (6 hour collection)

Fraction	Molecular weight	Dose (Mg)	Mg	%	Reference range
1	198	4.0	1.1	**28.2**	26.6–33.4
2	242	9.0	2.5	**28.2**	26.5–31.6
3	286	39.0	10.5	**27.0**	25.2–29.4
4	330	96.0	22.3	**23.2**	21.1–25.0
5	374	157.0	32.0	**20.4**	17.9–22.0
6	418	171.0	25.1	**14.7**	12.5–16.2
7	462	176.0	14.4	**8.2**	6.4–10.8
8	506	145.0	5.8	**4.0**	3.6–6.0
9	550	105.0	1.1	**1.0**	1.0–2.4
10	594	67.0	0.2	**0.3**	Up to 1.4
11	638	31.0	0.0	**0.0**	Up to 0.7
	TOTAL:	**1000.0**	**115.1**	**11.5**	**10.0–13.3%**

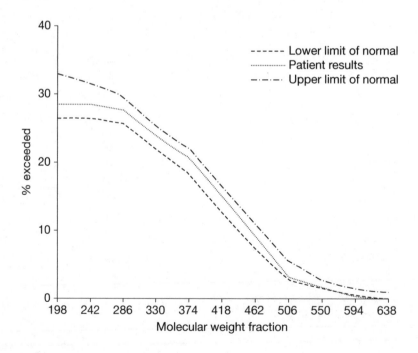

Figure 5.4ac: Typical profile for healthy individual

very small amount of the larger lactulose molecule is absorbed. However, the smaller molecules of mannitol are absorbed through the lining of the small intestine (the jejunum and duodenum). The two sugars are excreted via the urine and can be measured. The relative ratio of the two sugars is used to determine the increased gut-permeability (high levels of lactulose) or poor absorption (low levels of mannitol).

Comprehensive digestive stool analysis

Another test, this time offered by Genova Diagnostics, is the comprehensive digestive stool analysis. It evaluates digestion, absorption, gut flora and the state of the interior of the colon, including immunology. The profile is recommended for all those who have chronic gut problems, acute bowel pattern changes and many systemic diseases. It also provides a sensitivity panel for treating pathogenic flora.

The test requires two samples from one random stool. Any medication with antibiotics, anti-fungals or probiotics must be stopped at least two weeks beforehand. Some drugs may also compromise the accuracy of the results, including steroids, and non-steroid anti-inflammatory drugs (NSAIDs, such as ibuprofen and aspirin).

The test can provide results for the following factors:

Beneficial flora (*Bifidobacterium, Escherichia coli, Lactobacillus*)

Imbalanced and dysbiotic flora

Bacteriology enzyme immune assay (EIA) (*Campylobacter pylori*, Shiga-like toxin, *E coli*)

Mycology

Mucus

Occult blood

Chymotrypsin

Putrefactive short-chain fatty acids

Meat fibres

Vegetable fibres

Triglycerides

Long-chain fatty acids

Cholesterol

Phospholipids

Total faecal fat

Faecal lactoferrin

Beneficial short-chain fatty acids

n-Butyrate

beta-Glucuronidase

pH

Acetate

Proprionate

Colour

Anti-microbial sensitivities

In addition, prescription and natural agents can be tested on an individual basis.

Glucose tolerance testing

My first book, *Low Blood Sugar*, was published, in 1981. It had the subtitle *The 20th Century Epidemic?* Prior to this book, low blood sugar (hypoglycaemia) was viewed by medicine as a harmless and transient symptom, resulting from a missed meal, acute stress or one of several symptoms occurring with the pre-menstrual syndrome. A rather more serious known cause was miss-judged insulin dosage, occurring occasionally with type I diabetes.

To quote a passage from my book:

'The chance observations of an obscure American doctor in the 1920s led to the discovery that reactive hypoglycaemia is an important cause of a great variety of symptoms. Seale Harris was a general practitioner living in the state of Alabama and a contemporary of Banting and Best, the co-discoverers of the role of insulin in diabetes. Harris noticed that many diabetic patients attending the new insulin clinics developed symptoms of low blood sugar. This paradox is not difficult to understand if you see insulin and sugar as being at opposite ends of the scale. When there is balance the scale is level, but if one is in excess, the other is deficient. Many diabetics have difficulty in accurately judging their insulin requirements and often overdose themselves, producing a condition known as hyperinsulinism which consequently causes hypoglycaemia. This "hypo" or insulin effect is characterised by symptoms of anxiety, fatigue, breathlessness and palpitations. Essentially the diabetic has swung from high to low blood sugar due to an inappropriate increase in the blood insulin level. Fortunately, this is a transient effect. Most diabetics learn to avoid the "hypo" situation by carefully balancing their insulin dosage, diet and energy output, at the same time regularly monitoring their blood and urine sugar levels.'

To return to Dr Harris, he noted that he had in his practice several patients who exhibited symptoms of the 'hypo' reaction on a regular basis, but who were *not* diabetic and who were, therefore, not taking insulin. He accurately concluded that these patients probably experienced the unpleasant symptoms of hypoglycaemia as a result of overactivity or imbalance in their insulin-producing apparatus. This complex mechanism involves the islet glands of the pancreas, the liver, to some extent the pituitary, thyroid and adrenal glands and many other factors which play their part in sugar metabolism.

In 1924 Seale Harris presented his theories in a paper published in the *Journal of the American Medical Association*. His reasoning on the possible causes of hypoglycaemia in non-diabetic patients led him to conclude that many glands of the body can be 'hypo' or 'hyper' active and that frequently underactivity (hypo) is preceded by overactivity (hyper). This concept is not difficult to appreciate as overactivity, with subsequent exhaustion or damage, is a characteristic of many organs and systems within the body. Any overworked machine usually malfunctions.

Dr Harris discussed his ideas with Dr Banting (the co-discoverer of insulin metabolism), who agreed that the role of insulin in hypoglycaemia offered a new aspect to the study of blood sugar balance, presenting a mirror image to the diabetic situation. No papers on this topic had appeared in medical literature prior to Seale Harris's historic work, but his discoveries led to a glut of similar papers in journals all over the world.

The American *Annals of Internal Medicine* included a further paper by Harris in 1936. This definitive statement precisely classified the causes and symptoms of hypoglycaemia. Although subsequent research has shown that the relationship of low blood sugar to excess insulin in the blood is not so simplistic as defined by Harris, it is now recognised that the whole glandular system is involved in our blood sugar balance.

The six-hour glucose tolerance test

You may be familiar with the two-hour glucose tolerance test that is used to diagnose diabetes. While useful for that purpose, it is virtually valueless for establishing reactive hypoglycaemia as the important 'over swing' (rapid drop in blood glucose) occurs after more than two hours. The six-hour glucose tolerance test is the most reliable test for reactive hypoglycaemia and is usually referred to as the 'GTT'. However, it is only valid if the following conditions are met:

1. It is combined with a physical examination
2. The test is preceded by noting down a detailed case history
3. The patient has described and listed his/her own diet and symptoms
4. The patient's reactions and symptoms during the test are noted and timed
5. The glucose dosage and the timing of blood sampling are standardised for every test
6. No dramatic changes have recently been made to the patient's diet
7. The physician is fully aware of any drugs being taken by the patient.

It must be remembered that some hypoglycaemics do not show symptoms, while others show pronounced hypoglycaemic symptoms with a normal blood sugar level. This is why it is essential to standardise the test procedures and to know each patient as thoroughly as possible before the test.

Test procedure

The patient is requested to fast for 12 hours (only water permitted), and to attend the surgery at 9 am. The fast is no great hardship as only breakfast is missed. Obviously it is important that no food or drink (except water) is taken until the test is completed at 3.30 pm.

During the course of the test, seven small blood samples are taken. The first sample, taken at 9.15 am, shows the level of fasting blood sugar (FBS), and is followed at 9.30 am by the drinking of 50 grams (2 ounces) of soluble glucose. The remaining six samples are then taken to monitor the effects of the glucose on the patient's blood sugar level over time.

The amount of glucose used in the GTT can vary, 100 grams (4 ounces) being the usual test dose in America. This higher dose can occasionally make the more sensitive patients nauseous or faint, and it is not normally used in the UK. (There is no available evidence to suggest that it improves diagnostic accuracy.)

The blood sugar level is constantly changing and, even with seven samples taken in six hours, one obtains only a guide to the dynamics of blood glucose activity. It is possible the highest reading may in fact lie *between* two samples. If I suspect that this has occurred and the speed of the patient's insulin response has been so rapid that the GTT has not confirmed a diagnosis, a repeat test is requested. This is a shorter version, also using 50 grams (2 ounces) of glucose, but with a blood sample taken every 15 minutes over a 1½ hour period. In this way the all-important upper figure is more precisely assessed. The sample times are obviously at the convenience of your practitioner. I find the following schedule most suitable.

```
Patient arrives ----------------- 9.00 am
Sample 1 FBS taken --------- 9.15 am
50 g glucose taken ------------ 9.30am
Sample 2 ---------------------- 10.00 am
Sample 3 ---------------------- 10.30 am
Sample 4 ---------------------- 11.30 am
Sample 5 -----------------------12.30 pm
Sample 6 ---------------------- 2.00 pm
Sample 7 ---------------------- 3.30 pm
```

This means that the samples are taken at the following times *after* drinking the glucose.

```
Sample 2 ------------------------ ½ hour
Sample 3 ------------------------ 1 hour
Sample 4 ------------------------2 hours
Sample 5 ------------------------3 hours
Sample 6 --------------------- 4½ hours
Sample 7 ------------------------6 hours
```

The patient is encouraged to remain active during the tests, keeping, if possible, within his/her own normal daily energy output, and is required at the surgery only for the sample-taking. (In case symptoms develop during the second half of the test when blood sugar is coming down, a restroom needs to be available.)

As many patients do not feel very alert after the completion of the test, they are advised to arrange for someone to drive them home. It is also sensible to have some bread and cheese or a glass of milk as soon as possible after the test has been completed.

Symptoms produced by the GTT

The symptoms that arise during the test and the timing of the onset of these symptoms are both of considerable diagnostic value. When the glucose readings are explained to the patient on his/her next visit, it is always interesting to note that the symptoms experienced during the test (such as nausea, headache, stomach pains, lethargy and dizziness) usually arise as the blood sugar falls. The majority of patients are quite impressed to learn that their symptoms, often attributed to stress or imagination, can be reproduced by the simple method of taking a glucose drink. For them, this confirms the diagnosis of hypoglycaemia in a far more tangible way than could a set of blood test results. This clinical confirmation of a puzzling condition is often very reassuring to the patient.

GTT results

This valuable test can establish a diagnosis of diabetes or hypoglycaemia. Although the orthodox medical view holds that reactive hypoglycaemia is a rare condition, the evidence points to the contrary. I have found that out of 201 patients selected and tested with a six-hour GTT, 92% showed clearly defined reactive hypoglycaemia.

Since Seale Harris first described hypoglycaemia in 1924, no single, generally accepted guideline defining this condition has been agreed upon. The GTT is open to various interpretations, depending on the doctor's view of what constitutes 'normal'. (As with many types of measurement used in medicine, the figures for the average patient cannot necessarily be taken as the norm!) Dr Harris stated that in his view a diagnosis of hypoglycaemia is justified if the GTT shows a blood sugar reading *below* the commonly accepted lower limit (that is, 4–6 mmol/l).This, he insisted, must be supported by the reproduction of hypoglycaemic symptoms during the course of the test. Over the intervening years the required lower limit, below which hypoglycaemia could be established, has been reduced to 2.2 mmol/l. This rather rigid criterion for diagnosis has fortunately been modified in recent years, with the general recognition that each GTT result should be assessed in relation to the patient. An individual's response to the glucose drink should be observed in terms of speed of absorption, and speed of insulin response. A patient may have pronounced symptoms of hypoglycaemia yet show a set of glucose readings that are all within 'normal' limits. Close attention to symptoms before and during the GTT is of greater diagnostic value than slavish adherence to a set of normal ranges. I have seen patients experience distressing symptoms of hypoglycaemia when their blood sugar has fallen during a GTT from 8 mmol to 4 mmol, the symptoms being caused not by the *level* of glucose but by the inappropriate *speed* of the fall.

To understand what is happening in the GTT it may be helpful to discuss the *normal* result, before going further, and the manner in which it is presented. A normal set of results is shown in table 5.1.

Table 5.1: Normal six-hour GTT result			
Sample	*Interval from 0 in hours*	*Time*	*Result in mmol/l*
1	0 (FBS)	9.15 am	4.5
	(50g glucose solution)	(9.30 am)	
2	½	10.00 am	7.8
3	1	10.30 am	7.2
4	2	11.30 am	4.8
5	3	12.30 pm	4.0
6	4½	2.00 pm	4.2
7	6	3.30 pm	4.5

As you can see, when the patient has taken the glucose, the blood sugar level rises (samples 2 and 3). As the glucose is absorbed, insulin is automatically released to control the rising blood sugar. With a normal insulin response, only an optimum amount of insulin is released, allowing the blood sugar level to fall to the individual's fasting level (sample 7). The results are plotted on a graph, producing a 'glucose tolerance curve'. One learns to recognise different types of curves; the configuration of a curve is diagnostically as important as the actual figures producing it.

Diagnosis using the GTT

When presented with a set of figures for a GTT, your practitioner's first step is to look for a possible diabetic component. A fasting level in excess of 7 mmol/l is strongly suggestive of diabetes, but some diabetics can have a fasting level under 6 mmol/l. For this reason, an assessment of the sum of the first four results obtained in the GTT is recommended by Dr Danowski of Pittsburg, as a more reliable method of identifying diabetes. If the *total* for the four samples is between 28 and 44 mmol/l, diabetes is suspected; if over 44 mmol/l, diabetes is positively confirmed.

There are many different types of GTT curve, for the dynamics of the blood sugar level are expressed in many ways. As stated, the actual level of blood sugar is related to symptoms during the test, but even more important is, perhaps, the speed at which the blood sugar responds to the insulin. A drop of from 7 mmol/l to 3.5 mmol/l in one hour may be more significant than a drop from 7 mmol/l to 2.2 mmol/l in two hours. The time taken for the sugar to return to a normal level (usually called the 'recovery'), and how long it remains at a low level, are also important diagnostic clues. For example, a fall to 2.2 mmol/l with a rapid recovery to normal may be less significant than a fall to 3.5 mmol/l that stays at this level for two to three hours before recovery.

It is very unusual to find any two GTT curves that are alike. So-called 'normal' values are based on population averages and may not reflect what is normal for the patient being tested.

Some disagreement surrounds the value of interpreting the 'fall' in blood sugar during the test. This represents the difference between the initial fasting level, and the lowest figure to which the blood sugar drops during the test. Dr Robert Atkins (of the *Atkins' Diet*) considers a 2 mmol/l drop essential before a conclusive diagnosis of hypoglycaemia can be given, whilst Carlton Fredericks (an authority on many aspects of nutrition and the author of *Low Blood Sugar and You* with H Goodman) finds a drop of between 0.8 mmol/l and 1 mmol/l to be sufficient. Other authorities (such as Dr Michael Somgyi) have set the figures of 0.2 to 0.3 mmol as diagnostically significant. These figures are, however, meaningful only within the context of symptoms arising during the test and an individual's reaction to the 50 grams (2 ounces) of glucose. I find in practice that a fall as small as 0.3 mmol/l can be associated with hypoglycaemic symptoms.

To conclude this description of the GTT, it may be worth quoting Carlton Fredericks. He states that, 'When blood sugar drops as little as 0.18 mmol below the normal for the patient, a profound glandular compensation may start.' In his view, no practitioner should disregard a blood sugar reading that is 'only a few points below normal', and if there is doubt, a diagnosis of hypoglycaemia with correct treatment should be considered.

Glucometers

A glucometer allows one accurately to measure one's blood glucose with a single finger-prick of blood in 3–4 seconds. As they are readily available and low cost (around £12–£15 from most chemists), I like to recommend that patients do their own blood glucose measurements. They can, of course, follow the seven-sample six-hour GTT schedule after taking 50 grams of soluble glucose. Nevertheless, I tend to point out the value of testing when their symptoms arise, examples being: on rising, with missed meals, or when shaky, or with excessive yawning. For the ladies, pre-menstrual blood sugar checks can also be worthwhile.

So what levels could be considered as being abnormally low? Diabetic nurses have an expression: 'under four – on the floor', meaning if a glucose level below 4 mmol/l shows, then lie the patient down before he/she falls down. Such low glucose levels can cause irritability, pallor, confusion, yawning and eventual unconsciousness. I shall discuss this complex problem in greater detail in chapter 6, on treatment (see page 215). However, a diagnosis of low blood sugar points to a contributory cause of CFS, making it worth investigating.

How the naturopathic approach can contribute to the diagnosis and treatment of CFS

I think that I can safely say that alternative (or 'complementary', as I prefer) practitioners, naturopaths in particular, are rarely the first choice of exhausted patients seeking help. In my own practice, only around 10% of patients consult me before they consult their GP, often following a referral from a family member or partner. Comparisons are frequently made between mainstream medicine fronted by GPs and hospital consultants, and the alternative practitioners. These comparisons can be summarised as follows:

1. NHS doctors are restricted in the time permitted with each patient. Private doctors and alternative practitioners can usually allow more flexibility.
2. With the large-group GP practices within the NHS there cannot be a guarantee that the same doctor will be seen on every visit by each patient.
3. A GP's choice of tests is limited by available funding and the NHS laboratory test menu.

The NHS is Europe's largest employer. With such a huge organisation, the 'personal touch' is inevitably becoming a rarity. One outcome of this is that many medical doctors are choosing to leave the NHS to become private doctors. I have discussed this trend with GPs and found that the chief reason is a desire to be able to devote more time to their patients, and also to be able to specialise in particular areas of health that interest them. Unfortunately, those leaving the NHS tend to be the more competent GPs who the NHS can ill afford to lose.

As a registered naturopath, I am very conscious that private blood and other tests that are designed to identify the causes of CFS, and hopefully monitor a patient's progress, all need to be paid for. Harley Street is probably the most famous street in the world for practitioners of all therapies and I have seen patients in Harley Street over many years, the availability of the many specialised laboratories nearby being perhaps the chief benefit for those working in the area.

Regrettably, specialised testing that is not available via the NHS, with the addition of travel costs and treatment fees, can be beyond the budget of many CFS patients. This means that finding an ethical specialised practitioner who will not waste your time and money is of particular importance. If this practitioner can provide an accurate and personalised test selection and interpretation it will be of great value. You may well have travelled down numerous diagnostic cul-de-sacs already in your search for a healthier life-style. If you are looking for a naturopath to help you the register of qualified practitioners can be found at www.naturopathy.org.uk.

Chapter 6

The treatment of chronic fatigue syndrome

I hope after reading chapters 1 to 5 of this book you will agree that the chronic fatigue syndrome is a complex condition, with many potential, interrelated causes and therefore without a single, unitary cure. In other words, there is no 'magic bullet'. Because the complex of causes will be individual to each sufferer, there is no such thing as a common treatment strategy for CFS. The successful treatment can only result from detailed case-history taking, and accurate diagnosis based on a carefully selected range of tests, interpreted in the light of the sufferer's symptoms. I believe that an awareness of *all* the possible causes must be seen as an essential prerequisite for any successful treatment.

In the absence of a single, universally effective treatment for CFS, I tend to prefer a step-by-step approach to treatment.

As I said at the end of chapter 5, patients very rarely make naturopathy their first choice of treatment. Many people who consult me admit that they have previously sought a diagnosis and possible treatment for their CFS from a variety of practitioners. To confront yet another complete stranger is understandably distressing for any patient. I therefore have found that a systematic but personalised approach to case-history taking can be reassuring for new patients.

Diet

As a naturopath I consider that a detailed review of a new patient's diet is an essential first step. However, an appropriate ideal diet for CFS is much

143

disputed. The word 'controversial' is used to describe almost every aspect of CFS, including the definition, symptoms, diagnosis and treatment.

When one considers the enormous range of possible causes of chronic fatigue, the notion that there exists one ideal diet for all patients is very unrealistic. When patients request dietary advice from me, often on their first visit, I have a stock reply: 'I would like to find out more about your health before I recommend a diet.'

Many CFS sufferers have researched their symptoms via the internet, TV programmes and the press, sometimes over a period of several years. As a result they follow quite adequate diets. I talk to patients whose eating habits cannot be faulted in a general sense. Unfortunately, their diet is not always suited to their symptoms. Not surprisingly, they often express concern and annoyance that, in spite of all their efforts with food selection and 'healthy eating', they continue to be exhausted. I sometimes point to the analogy of a motor car that fails to start, even with high octane fuel.

Regrettably, quality food does not always guarantee quality health for CFS sufferers. Hence the frequent need to prescribe a customised diet. Many factors can influence food content, balance and priorities. There are many books available, whose authors advocate remedial diets for the treatment of all CFS suffferers. I will start by briefly reviewing these diets to emphasise the often contradictory advice offered.

Example 1

The medical advisor (in 2001) to the Chronic Fatigue and Immune Deficiency Association of America advised the following diet for CFS: 'Eat lots of complex carbohydrates. Avoid red meats and reduce the fats.' Fat, he claimed can 'sap your energy'. Recommended foods included: fruit, vegetables, bread and cereal, rice, pasta, chicken, turkey and fish.

Example 2

In the book *Fighting Fatigue*, by Sue Pemberton and Catherine Berry, the chapter on diet offers the following 'meal plan':

> Breakfast – bowl of wholemeal cereal, eg bran flakes, porridge with
> semi-skimmed milk or two slices of wholemeal bread spread with
> margarine/butter and jam.

Mid-morning – a drink and a banana/two oatcakes/wholemeal scone with jam/cereal bar.

Lunch – sandwich with two slices of wholemeal bread with a filling of your choice and a piece of fruit/ yoghurt.

Mid-afternoon – a drink and two oatcakes, fruit cake, piece of fruit/ handful of nuts/cereal bar.

Evening meal – wholemeal pasta/brown rice/jacket potato/basmati rice, with fish/meat/eggs/quorn/cheese and vegetables, plus pudding eg stewed fruit and custard/rice pudding/yoghurt.

Supper – piece of fruit/2 biscuits/dried fruit (small handful)/small chocolate bar/bowl of cereal.

The following advice is included: 'Carbohydrates are essential for energy and therefore should make up approximately 50–70% of your everyday diet.'

Example 3

Alison Adams, in her book *Chronic Fatigue, ME and Fibromyalgia*, advocates the following diet:

Meal	Options
Breakfast	Oatmeal or rice porridge, sugar-free or homemade muesli, unsweetened oat cereals, Boiled egg and oatcakes, fruit, scrambles eggs with smoked salmon, bacon, tomatoes and sautéed potatoes, brown rice kedgeree, buckwheat pancakes and berries, gluten-free cereal and rice milk.
Lunch	Meat, fish and/or vegetable soups, salads with chicken, fish or meat, rice salad, leftovers like casserole, sushi, baked potato with prawns (no mayonnaise), tuna or homemade chilli, oatcakes with homemade fish pâté or cold meat, fruit or fruit salad.
Evening meal	Meat, poultry or fish with vegetables and homemade sauce or gravy, spelt or rice pasta, with homemade sauce, chicken, prawn or meat stir-fry, with rice or rice noodles, risotto, homemade curry with rice, casserole or stew and potatoes.

Drink advice is not included in this diet.

On comparing these three examples, your initial question may be, why is there such a wide variety of recommended foods across the three diets? There seems to be no general theme in the regimes and no common pattern. There is, however, one shared concept: the emphasis on the value of carbohydrates. (You will have noted that Alison Adams advises up to 70% of the diet should consist of carbohydrates.) Although all the authors emphasise the need for the carbohydrates to be 'wholegrain or wholemeal', there is evidence that wholemeal and refined (white flour, rice etc) products have a similar effect on our blood sugar metabolism. It has been said by many authorities that, 'colour doesn't matter'.

The variations in these regimes serve to highlight the difficulties involved in attempting to design an all-purpose diet for CFS. As I have stated earlier in this chapter, I find that diets for CFS sufferers usually need to be customised to the person's state of health and nutritional requirements; their symptoms are often a result of nutritional deficiencies. Specific health problems that contribute to CFS symptoms, including candidiasis, leaky gut syndrome, iron and vitamin B-12 deficiencies, obesity and syndrome X, may require tailored diets. To illustrate this need to customise, each section in this chapter includes a case history, many of which include a specific diet to match and treat the individual's symptoms.

I must add that I have yet to see a severely exhausted CFS patient fully recover with diet change alone. Many such people have, of their own accord, dabbled with a range of different self-prescribed diets in the hope of some symptom relief. Actual improvement with such diets is regrettably minimal. Nevertheless, a degree of relief from the many symptoms under the CFS umbrella can be achieved with elimination diets, rotation diets, effective weight loss diets, low-carbohydrate diets and many others. Unfortunately, any symptom-relief often tends to be transient, leading patients to attempt a succession of varying programmes with little long-term benefit.

A healthy diet
This seems to be an ideal point to describe what I believe to be a good, healthy diet. The purpose of this diet is to emphasise food priorities and choice, but

also to draw attention to the foods and drinks that need to be limited, or in some cases avoided, if the diet is to be nutritious, enjoyable and effective. There are two main aims for this diet:

1. Weight control
2. Blood sugar control

These two objectives are best achieved with a very low-carbohydrate diet, which contrasts with the three examples I have quoted. It also contrasts with current medical recommendations for the ideal daily food group proportions. The *Merck Manual*, the medical 'bible' for medical information, advises the food proportions shown in Figure 6.1.

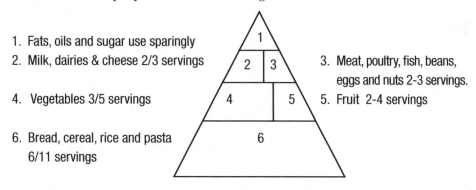

1. Fats, oils and sugar use sparingly
2. Milk, dairies & cheese 2/3 servings
3. Meat, poultry, fish, beans, eggs and nuts 2-3 servings.
4. Vegetables 3/5 servings
5. Fruit 2-4 servings
6. Bread, cereal, rice and pasta 6/11 servings

Figure 6.1: Food guide pyramid showing recommended daily servings

The low-carbohydrate diet

History and value

Long before Dr Robert Atkins designed and recommended his low-carbohydrate diet that became a popular choice for the overweight, many other similar diets had been advocated. In 1905 an Australian physician, Francis Hare, who became the Inspector General of hospitals in Queensland, wrote a massive 1000-page, two-volume book entitled *The Food Factor in Disease*. The second volume included 86 detailed case histories, describing his patients, suffering from migraine, asthma, arthritis, anaemia, fatigue and many other problems. A symptom common for many of his patients was 'debility', the word he used to describe fatigue and defined in the book as 'lack or loss of strength'.

The diets prescribed by Dr Hare were all low in carbohydrates, with fat and protein at every meal and no sugar. Fruit and root vegetables were reduced, or even forbidden to some patients. For interest, here are two typical case histories:

Case 1: Dr Hare described a young, underweight woman with fatigue, headaches, acne and scanty periods; she was aged 22 and weighed 6½ stone. Her diet consisted mainly of carbohydrates. Treatment was by diet only, as follows: meat, fish or eggs were insisted upon at each of her three meals; starch foods were cut down to three ounces daily and sugar excluded. She also had a pint and a half of milk daily. Her symptoms had improved in all areas within four weeks and her weight had increased by four pounds, her skin problems having disappeared and her energy improved.

Case 2: This was a woman aged 30 years. To quote Dr Hare: 'On arrival, she was fat, flabby, anaemic and extremely weak, hardly able to walk indeed. Her special affliction was recurrent gastralgia, coming on once a week with intense pain, and nausea.' The treatment was a diet that only included lean meat and milk. The quantities were 'left to the patient'. At the end of the fortnight, she was taking meat three times daily, together with eight pints of milk, taken little and often. After four weeks she was allowed a little bread and butter. To quote Dr Hare again: 'The result was immediate cessation of the gastralgic attacks and a progressive increase in strength. Her colour returned and she enjoyed better health than ever before in her life.'

So what do we learn from this 108-year-old book that describes patients in the late 19th century who all followed a low-carbohydrate programme? The first obvious conclusion is that there is nothing new about CFS. There is also nothing new about the trendy low-starch diets that have been named after enthusiastic practitioners and made the subjects of popular medicine books. The concept of the curative value of fat and protein is also not a recent issue, and the overrated importance of five to six potions of fruit and vegetables daily is clearly questionable.

As a 21st-century naturopath, I can see the need for a little nutritional fine-tuning with Dr Hare's diets. However, his book constitutes an early master class in the effective treatment of many health problems, without recourse to the current emphasis in mainstream medicine on high-carbohydrate eating.

Chapter 6

You may be wondering, what do I mean by 'nutritional fine-tuning'? The best way to answer is to describe the low-carbohydrate diet that I regularly prescribe for a variety of health problems.

The Martin Budd low-carbohydrate diet
Breakfast

The most important meal of the day following a 10- to 12-hour night-fast
Avoid bread, cereal and also muesli

Cold

Can include cold ham and meats, cheese, pâté, smoked fish, hard-boiled eggs, sardines etc

Hot

Eggs (scrambled, poached, boiled, as an omelette or fried with unsalted butter)
Grilled or steamed fish
Tomatoes, mushrooms and cheese
Smoked fish, eg kippers or mackerel
When frying, clarified butter or lard are best
Pure oils, eg sunflower, olive and blended cooking oils, are all unsuitable for cooking at high temperatures (frying) and olive oil tends to flavour the food

Drink

Natural yoghurts, raw milk, water or coffee

Lunch

First choice (cold)

Salad, meat, fish, cheese or eggs with plenty of lettuce and tomatoes etc; use French dressing
Avoid potato salad, pasta and bread

Second choice (hot)

Protein can include (as Dinner) eggs, fish, meat, poultry, game
Hot meal but *avoid* potatoes, pasta, pastry, rice and bread
Plenty of green vegetables
For dessert have cheese without bread or biscuits

Third choice

Sandwiches (starch-reduced bread): maximum two slices of bread, with plenty of butter; contents can include cheese, beef, ham and chicken slices

Cods' roes and cooked white fish

Salmon or tuna (avoiding tinned fish with added sugar)

Cheese with tomatoes, sliced onions or ham

Drink

Dry wine (one glass) or water, raw milk and natural yoghurts

(Raw milk is widely available on the continent, customers being allowed to fill their own containers in supermarkets with milk direct from the farm. It is only available in England and Wales bought direct from farms, online and at farmers' markets. In Scotland its sale is banned outright.)

Dinner

Typical cooked meal but *avoid* potatoes, pasta, pastry, rice and bread; compensate by eating extra eggs, fish, meat, cheese, poultry and game. (It is important to include animal fat and poultry skin)

Root vegetables

Approximately 1 cupful when chopped

Green vegetables

Unlimited, as appetite allows

Drink

Water, dry wine (one glass)

Try to drink 2 pints (8 glasses) of water each day; avoid tap water unless filtered

Drinking before meals is recommended (15–20 minutes before)

Fruit

Limit fruit to *one* portion daily (or exclude with proven gut fermentation conditions)

Fruit has been defined as 'nature's candy' as a result of the fructose content

Chapter 6

Snacks

Can include 1 ounce of sunflower seeds or nuts (walnut, brazil, peanut, cashew etc)

Fibre can be found in *all* plant foods

An ideal food groups ratio is: carbohydrates – 10% maximum; protein – 25% minimum; fat – 65% minimum

NB The human need for carbohydrates is *nil*.

Important note This diet should be used only when under the direct supervision of the practitioner.

Low-carbohydrate diets – a review

As I have previously described, Dr Atkins's diet and his books were preceded by other practitioners' diets and other books. In the last century, such a diet was advocated to treat diabetics, before insulin was discovered in the 1930s. William Banting, John Yudkin, T I Cleave, Richard Mackarness, Charles Clark, Michael Eades, Herman Tannower (Scarsdale Diet) and Barry Groves have all recommended similar diets. Why then is the diet so controversial? The arguments tend to hinge on the fats versus carbohydrate conflict.

When mankind was a nomadic hunter-gatherer species around 10,000 years ago, the basic diet was high in protein and fat with occasional seeds, nuts and roots. With the gradual development of agriculture and the storage of grain, the hunters became farmers and by necessity lived in fixed settlements. The swing from animal protein and fat to root crops and cereals, with their relative deficiency in proteins, vitamins and minerals, led to a rise in nutritional deficiency diseases such as pellagra (vitamin B-3 deficiency), obesity, allergies, cancer, beriberi (vitamin B-1 deficiency), rickets and the many other 'diseases of civilisation'.

The processing of sugar was another blow to human health. The production of sugar from cane and beet causes loss of fibre, proteins, vitamins and minerals. The pure 'sucrose' that remains at the end of the process actually requires vitamins for its metabolism. Sugar consumption in the UK 200 years ago was around 2 kilograms (4 pounds) per person per year. The figure is now 60 kilograms (130 pounds) per person per year.

151

Examples of a 'primitive' diet could still be seen in action up to 50 years ago. The Eskimos of Greenland existed almost entirely on mostly raw fish and meat. The Maasai herdsmen of East Africa only consumed the blood, milk and occasional meat from their cattle. Unfortunately, the diets of both groups have become 'civilised' and subsequently richer in carbohydrates. Their health has deteriorated as a result.

Fat versus sugar

It is unfortunate that the word we use to describe an overweight person is the same word used to define a major and very essential food group; the word of course is 'fat'. We would never refer to an obese person as 'too sugary'; we always say 'too fat'. Consequently, the link between fat in food and people becoming fat is now well established in most people's minds.

Calorie counting – the background

Calorie counting has been the basis of diet design for many years. The calorific content of food groups is as follows:

A gram of carbohydrate provides 4.2 calories
A gram of protein provides 4.25 calories
A gram of fat provides 9.2 calories.

These calorific levels are used to indicate the energy value of foods and to enable slimmers to measure their food intake. You will immediately note why low-fat diets are so popular; fat provides more than twice the calories of proteins and carbohydrates. The thinking behind calorie counting is, however, flawed.

Calorie counting – the flaws

The calorie is a heat unit. The heat given off when a measured amount of food is burnt (in a calorimeter) is called its calorific value. However, many naturopaths and nutritionists believe that calorie counting, as a basis for weight loss, is a waste of time and effort. These are the reasons why:

1. The human body is *not* a calorimeter, simply converting food to energy. We lose a lot of energy when we digest food; an example is the formation of ketones, which are eliminated via the kidneys, when excess fat is consumed. Ketones have a calorific value of around 4 calories per gram, thus reducing the calorific value of fat. (A diet that leads to ketone formation is termed 'ketogenic'.)

2. The total calorie count for any diet offers a guide to food quantity but not food quality, nor the metabolic effect of the diet. A low-carbohydrate 2000-calorie diet may persuade your metabolism to utilise fat in place of sugar (carbohydrate) for energy and require less insulin to be produced. Thus you lose weight. However, a low-fat, high-carbohydrate diet of 2000 calories may cause you to gain weight. One advantage of a low-carbohydrate diet is that burning the fat in your diet takes more energy, and therefore uses more calories. So you will burn more calories yet experience less hunger when your body is fuelled with a low-carbohydrate, fat- and protein-based regime.

3. Food is not used simply for energy. We need protein for body tissue repair and maintenance (skin, hair, blood etc). Fats are also used to manufacture hormones and bile salts. The essential fatty acids are needed for the nervous system and brain. These basic needs account for a great many of the calories that are not used for energy. An example is the protein needed by a 12-stone (168 pounds or 76 kilogram) man for repair and maintenance alone, is equivalent to around 500 calories a day. Thus, to attempt to assess how many calories our bodies will store as fat when using a calorific diet is unsatisfactory and pointless.

Why avoid carbohydrate?

Unfortunately carbohydrate (sugar-rich) foods tend to be inexpensive, filling and tasty. All carbohydrates convert into sugar (glucose), but sugar is nutritionally bankrupt. Many low-fat recipes and products contain added sugar to improve flavour. Sugar when consumed requires insulin. The role of insulin is to convert the excess sugar in the blood into fat for storage, hence insulin is often termed the 'fattening hormone'. With a high-carbohydrate diet, the insulin becomes less and less effective ('insulin resistance'), prompting the body to produce more and more of it in order to metabolise the high sugar load, until finally the pancreas gives up, exhausted. Insulin resistance is the cause of many health problems.

Hypoglycaemia (low blood sugar)

When there is a high level of insulin in the blood, the intake of sugar can lead to a subsequent rapid fall in the blood sugar. This can cause dizziness, tremors, headache, anxiety and sugar craving. Those who overdose on sugar-rich carbohydrates suffer in a similar way to caffeine and alcohol addicts, where a vicious circle is maintained and frequently nutritious foods are excluded. Complex carbohydrates (in fruit and vegetables) are metabolised more slowly than carbohydrates from cereals and sugar and do not place such a strain on the insulin/glucose control. For this reason, any carbohydrates in your diet are best purchased from greengrocers and not from bakers, confectioners or grocers.

Low-carbohydrate diets – your questions and doubts answered

The low-carbohydrate approach, with its emphasis on fat and protein, has received a great deal of criticism. These are the chief concerns about such a diet, to which I offer answers:

1. **Avoiding carbohydrates leads to excess fat in the diet and high cholesterol**

   Answer: Cholesterol is an essential component of our body cell walls. It is used by our metabolism to make hormones, and bile salts. Only 20% of our total cholesterol is from food; the remaining 80% is manufactured in our livers. In scientific trials looking at diets that allowed unrestricted protein and fat, the so-called 'good' cholesterol (HDL) increased and the blood fat (triglycerides) reduced. Furthermore, the 'bad' cholesterol (LDL) did not increase.

2. **Eating fat in place of carbohydrates can cause ketosis**

   Answer: The chief 'fuel' produced from carbohydrate metabolism is glucose. In the usual so-called 'balanced' western diet, glucose provides most of the energy. We do, however, have a secondary fuel system using stored fat, with energy being provided from ketones. These are quite normal products of fat metabolism and their presence in the blood is termed 'ketosis'. Ketosis occurs in those who cannot use glucose for energy (for example, diabetics, anorexics, people who are starving and alcoholics). There is no evidence that ketones can increase to dangerous levels when you are following a very low-carbohydrate diet. With such a diet the blood ketones are usually the same on the second day as they are in the second month. Ketones can be excreted via the breath and in the urine, hence there is a need to drink plenty of water. Studies have confirmed that mild ketosis is harmless and will not increase to harmful levels in the blood of healthy dieters.

3. **Avoiding sugar-rich carbohydrates causes fatigue and constipation**
   Answer: Constipation may occur with a low-carbohydrate diet when fruit and vegetables are also avoided. Fibre is contained in all plant foods. These are an essential component of an effective diet. Any fatigue is only transient, rarely lasting longer than two to three days. The whole point of the diet is to change our body fuel from sugar to fat and our metabolism needs time to adapt to such a change.

4. **A high-protein low-carbohydrate diet can cause kidney damage and disease**
   Answer: There is no evidence based on specific cases or studies to support the view that a high-protein diet can lead to kidney damage. However, when someone is already suffering chronic advanced kidney disease, they are unlikely to be able to metabolise protein efficiently. When this occurs, a high-protein diet is inappropriate; such a diet is not, however, the cause of kidney disease or damage.

Health benefits of a low-carbohydrate diet

When discussing, reading about, or actually following a low-carbohydrate diet, the chief motivation and interest are weight loss. However, a diet that virtually avoids carbohydrate and recommends proteins and fats with each meal has many other health benefits.

Cholesterol, triglycerides and insulin – Detailed studies published in the *New England Journal of Medicine* in 2003 showed that when compared with a conventional high-carbohydrate, low-fat diet, the carbohydrate-avoidance diet led to a significant reduction in blood fat (triglycerides) and an increase in the 'good' cholesterol (HDL). Improvements in insulin sensitivity (the opposite of resistance) and weight loss were also predictable results of the low-carbohydrate diet. Meanwhile, the famous Framingham Heart Study was begun in Massachusetts in 1948 in an attempt to confirm that cholesterol-rich foods caused high blood cholesterol and subsequent heart disease and strokes. To the surprise of the researchers, those on high-fat diets experienced fewer strokes and lower cholesterol than those who followed a low-fat diet.

High blood pressure – The low-carbohydrate diet has a strong influence in lowering blood pressure, and those who take hypertensive drugs may need to adjust the dosage as their drug requirements reduce.

Diabetes – When type I and type II diabetics reduce their carbohydrates they will usually require less insulin or drugs to control their blood sugar. Therefore, as with hypertensive drugs and diuretics, you should keep your doctor informed of any diet change and request regular checks so that dependency on the drugs and insulin can be reduced.

Low blood sugar (hypoglycaemia) – Insulin resistance causes low blood sugar. Reducing carbohydrate and eating more fat and protein-rich foods serves to stabilise our blood sugar. This type of diet is therefore ideal for treating low blood sugar. The only special requirement when treating hypoglycaemia, in addition to my standard low-carbohydrate diet as outlined above (see page 149), is the need for four to five smaller meals each day to successfully control the low blood sugar.

Food combining – mirroring the Hay diet – The central component of the Hay diet is the need to avoid eating proteins and carbohydrates at the same meal (see below, page 162). The low-carbohydrate diet virtually excludes carbohydrates, making it an ideal equivalent to a food-combining diet. The benefits of food-combining diets include improved digestion, weight control and better health and vitality, which can all also be achieved with the low-carbohydrate diet.

Low-carbohydrate diets – summary
Unlike many similar diets, calorie counting and the exact carbohydrate content of
your meals and menus is not essential. Very reduced amounts of carbohydrates
are allowed in fruit and vegetables (see the diet for guidance, page 149). In
addition, particularly when weight targets have been achieved, organic Melba
toast, organic wholemeal crispbread, wheaten crackers and starch-reduced
bread can be introduced to add variety and additional fibre to the diet.

Nutritional approaches to CFS

The question of specific diets for specific health problems will surface several
times in this chapter, as you might expect. The treatments described for the
principal causes of CFS are backed by case histories, which usually include
prescribed diets. You will observe that I have in places repeated myself on
certain topics. I hope you will view this as the need for emphasis in preference
to memory lapses.

The bulk of this chapter covers treatment strategies for the common
causes of CFS, as were described in chapter 3. The final section discusses
possible treatment for the less common, more obscure causes, described in
chapter 4. Many of these contributory causes of fatigue are not accessible to
individual treatment. Nonetheless, they are usually worth considering when
a diagnostic and treatment protocol needs to be established.

I have also included a section dealing with non-nutritional treatments for
CFS. Some of these are specific therapies (such as the Perrin technique), whilst
others (such as Pilates) are systems and treatments with a known value for
those who suffer from CFS. Although many of these routines and therapies
are principally seen to be of value for symptom relief, they can contribute to
an overall programme to improve the recovery timescale for CFS patients.

Having described a review of a patient's diet as an essential first step in
treating chronic fatigue, I shall now add a few 'ifs' and 'buts' to the discussion.

Food choice and quality
The value of choosing, where possible, locally grown or produced food has
been much reviewed and generally agreed upon in recent years. We all have

access to news items, television programmes, magazine articles and, for many of us, internet information on this subject. The value and availability of local, seasonal produce have been discussed at length. Many authors in Europe and America have written controversial books covering such subjects as poor food quality, food commercialisation, food additives, pressure advertising and many other contentious topics. A selection of my favourite authors includes: Michael Moss, Bee Wilson, John Humphreys, Ben Goldacre, Barry Groves, Stanley Feldman with Vincent Marks, and Eric Schlosser.

Meanwhile our chefs and celebrity cooks have made us more aware of our poor quality school meals (Jamie Oliver), the use of country produce (Hugh Fearnley-Whittingstall), or simply good quality food and healthy cooking methods (Gary Rhodes, Nigel Slater, Simon Hopkinson etc). Having scanned today's main TV channels (Free-Sat) today being a typical quiet Thursday in March, I have identified 13 programmes whose subject matter is cooking or food. This does not include the radio programmes.

With such unrelenting advice on food selection, preparation and cooking it is difficult to believe that an unhealthy diet is possible in the UK. Although media and governmental advice on 'healthy' eating can be conflicting, we are all aware that refined, processed and generally harmful 'junk food' is best avoided. At the same time, I frequently encounter patients who admit that their diets are dreadful; their excuses range from lack of time to dislike of cooking or shopping, or simply a result of craving all the wrong foods.

Regrettably, a major motivation for many people's food selection is a result of economic necessity. Such items as convenience foods, TV snacks, cakes, biscuits, crisps, chocolate, cola-drinks and alcohol feature as essential components in many weekly housekeeping bills. Quality proteins, in particular beef and fish, are beyond the household budgets of many families. The failure of many schools to give basic education in cookery is also very much to blame. It would be so easy for all teenagers (both sexes) to have basic cookery skills taught to them whilst at school, to form a basis upon which to draw in their adult life. It is common knowledge that many school children do not know where milk, eggs and common vegetables (potatoes, tomatoes etc) have come from, or how they are grown.

I have already outlined my opposition to high-carbohydrate diets and criticised the 'healthy eating' maxim that advocates five portions of fruit and vegetables daily. Such disorders as syndrome X, diabetes, obesity and a huge range of health problems can result from such diets. I have emphasised the value of eating proteins at each meal and also animal fats as part of a recommended diet. There is only one advantage to a high-carbohydrate diet: it is inexpensive. A diet rich in cereal foods and root vegetables has been defined as 'peasant food'. Protein foods have for centuries been the preferred food of the middle and upper classes. One only has to look at the favoured food of different countries and cultures to identify this class bias. Obvious examples of 'people's foods' are rice in China, cereals and pulses in India, pasta in the Mediterranean area, wheat in Europe and America and potatoes in Ireland. Carbohydrates are cheap, filling, tasty and usually easy to prepare.

This has made the current official recommendation for the diet to consist of 50–70% carbohydrates all the easier for people to adopt. However, it is seen by many as a major cause of the obesity, diabetes and heart disease epidemics that afflict the so-called civilised nations. Perhaps CFS should be added to the above list; certainly the prevalence of chronic fatigue, with the often related symptom of depression, is increasing each year.

The treatment of many health problems requires nutritional intervention and advice. Problems that are directly food related include gastro-intestinal complaints, leaky gut, candidiasis and food allergies, but systemic general health problems may also benefit from this approach.

Food digestion

Having reviewed the relative value of fresh, locally produced food versus processed 'junk' food, the next topic must be the part digestion plays in the breakdown of our health.

I want to start by considering several, generally held misconceptions concerning our digestion:

1. It doesn't matter what we eat, as rubbish is eliminated and all the nutrients are absorbed.
2. The typical symptoms of indigestion – such as stomach fullness and wind, diarrhoea and/or constipation, heartburn and nausea – are all transient symptoms resulting from hurried meals or stress and are not serious health disorders.

3. The symptoms of indigestion can usually be solved by ant-acids, Immodium, paracetamol and other self-prescribed medicines. Advice or treatment is rarely necessary.

These misconceptions may be reassuring, but they prevent us from seeing what the problems really are. Digestive disorders, as with many ailments, do not always present matching symptoms. Achlorydria (lack of stomach acid), reduced pancreatic enzyme status, leaky gut, and low short-chain fatty acid levels do not present predictable diagnosable symptoms. To put it simply, a lot can go wrong before you are aware of the problem. This can result in a situation where quite serious gut problems can develop over several years before real action is taken to accurately diagnose and effectively treat the condition. I have a patient who had been prescribed ant-acids for eight years, for an acid stomach, before a gastroscopy was requested and a stomach tumour diagnosed. This resulted in surgery to remove one third of his stomach, yet this life-saving emergency surgery was preceded only by occasional heartburn and nausea until a few days before the stomach operation, when he developed severe blood loss and black stools. Not surprisingly, he had no awareness of the potential seriousness of his condition.

The gastro-intestinal tract is vital for energy production for our entire metabolism. The efficiency of every body organ can be compromised by digestive disorders.

Naturopathic medicine, or 'functional medicine' as it has been termed in America, has promoted many clinical approaches designed to treat gastro-intestinal disorders. A brief review of these diets and treatment methods will serve to emphasise the value of the drug-free systems that have been prescribed to normalise gut function. I do not endorse all of these regimes, but I do agree with the common theme of non-invasive therapies to treat indigestion, without recourse to drug-based symptom relief.

Diets to treat digestive conditions

Macrobiotic diets

'Macrobiotics' were originally conceived as a dietary concept around 200 years ago by C W Hufeland, a German professor. He recommended the consumption of plant foods that were native to the patient's location. The diet was developed under the eastern Yin-Yang philosophy, 'Yin' foods being leafy foods and fruit and 'Yang' foods being derived from stems, roots and seeds. Consequently, Yang foods were suitable for cold regions and Yin foods for hotter regions. The Japanese variation of the macrobiotic diet includes sea food. This is a simple and effective diet that needs care with ensuring sufficient essential nutrients, especially proteins, are included.

Vegetarian and vegan diets

Vegetarian and vegan diets are a constant source of controversy amongst dieticians, nutritionists, doctors and naturopaths, the key areas of dispute being plant versus animal protein and the possible tendency for those following such diets to develop vitamin B-12, zinc and ferritin deficiencies as a result of avoiding red meat. Vegetarians and vegans point to the availability of many plant proteins. In his book *Mental and Elemental Nutrients*, Carl Pfeiffer makes the valid observation that with careful planning and preparation, a vegetarian diet can be perfectly adequate to maintain health. Properly designed vegetarian diets can work well; several of my practitioner colleagues are strict and very healthy vegetarians. I am not convinced, however, that a vegan programme can work as well. The main non-meat protein option in such a diet is soya, yet another controversial choice.

I have discussed the merits and shortcomings of vegetarian and vegan diets with many CFS patients. Those who follow such diets are particularly vulnerable to three key health problems: vitamin B-12 deficiency, ferritin (iron stores) deficiency and adrenal fatigue. I am not suggesting that everyone who chooses to avoid animal protein is likely to become anaemic or unduly stressed. Nonetheless, I have observed a characteristic sluggish response to treatment with such patients. This is not too difficult to comprehend, as red meat is our chief source of both iron and vitamin B-12 and our requirements for proteins in the diet tend to increase when we are under stress. Certainly, I find that recovery from CFS with meat-free diets can be slower and compromised without an aggressive supplement programme. I frequently resort to prescribing vitamin B-12 injections and specific iron supplements when needed. Reliance on dietary iron and vitamin B-12 food sources can prove to be inadequate.

The Hay diet (food-combining diet)

William Hay devised a dietary system based on the principle of acid-forming and alkali-forming foods. I quote from *Naturopathic Medicine* by Roger Newman-Turner: 'The Hay Diet, as it came to be known, advocates care in the combination of foods which require different conditions for their digestion. Proteins, for example, require acid solutions for their digestion, which starts in the stomach and continues in the intestines. Carbohydrates, however, require alkaline secretions, which begin in the mouth and continue in the intestines. A mixture of protein and starch in the same meal is therefore, contraindicated because it is maintained that one prevents the proper digestion of the other. Another incompatible combination is starch with acid fruit.

'Hay advocated a diet of 20% acid-forming and 80% alkali-forming foods, maintaining that the selection of compatible food categories in any single meal would prevent progressive acid saturation which leads to ill-health. Although this system was recommended as a way of eating on a permanent basis, it is also used therapeutically, in the management of gastro-intestinal disorders when incompatible food combinations can be an unnecessary stress on a poorly functioning digestive system.'

The Hay diet, although a logical approach to digestive problems is now rarely prescribed as it is difficult for people to follow.

The blood-type diet

An American naturopath called James D'Adamo observed, when he worked in European clinics, that while some patients responded well to the prescribed diets, others showed no improvement or in fact got worse. This led him to test the patients' blood types (groups). He found that patients with type O blood group were suited to animal proteins while those with type A were better on a vegetarian regime. His son, Peter D'Adamo, developed this theory further and found that diets that were individualised on the basis of patients' blood groups led to clinical improvement, for a huge range of illnesses. The system was based on the inter-reaction of specific proteins on the walls of blood cells with incompatibility causing adverse reactions.

Fasting

By definition, fasting is the voluntary avoidance of food, so it cannot be described as a diet. Although lengthy fasts were encouraged in naturopathic clinics and 'hydros', some years ago, the current recommended maximum period for fasting tends to be three to seven days. It is of value as a therapy to mobilise the body's self-healing and to stimulate beneficial metabolic change (see *Naturopathic Medicine* by Roger Newman-Turner).

Stone Age ('paleo') diet

The principle behind this diet is that evolutionarily we are suited to a 'hunter-gatherer' diet (meat, nuts, berries, leafy vegetables) and that our bodies have not had time to evolve properly to utilise grain (eaten only for the last 10,000 years) or refined carbohydrates (eaten only for the last 150 years). The diet therefore excludes common foods, including refined wheat products, milk, eggs and sugar. Devised by Richard McKarness in his book *Not All in the Mind*, the diet is very similar to the type of diet recommended for many years by naturopaths. It is not too different from my own low-carbohydrate diet described earlier in this chapter (see page 149).

The 4R programme

Any effective treatment protocol for gastro-intestinal disorders involves more than dietary advice. This particularly applies if there is evidence that the patient's breakdown, absorption and eventual elimination of food is in any way faulty or compromised by stomach acid imbalance, poor enzyme status, gut fermentation, gut toxins and bacteria and leaky gut, or other conditions. In the *Textbook of Functional Medicine*, published by the Institute of Functional Medicine in 2005, Dan Lukaczer, one of the contributing authors, described a method for improving gut function termed the '4R programme'. The four 'Rs' eluded to are: 'remove', 'replace', 'reinoculate' and 'repair'. This model provides a paradigm for the effective treatment of many imbalances, deficiencies and actual diseases that can cause gut symptoms.

Part 1 – Remove – This aspect of the programme advocates the elimination of bacteria, parasites, fungi and yeasts and any other toxic substances from the gastro-intestinal tract. This can also include foods which may be suspected of, or proven to be, causing symptoms. The role of food allergies and intolerances is much disputed in medicine. However, there is little doubt that food sensitivities do exist and can cause a range of symptoms.

Part 2 – Replace – This key element involves the replacement of digestive enzymes and hydrochloric acid, the intrinsic factor and bile. Two-phase supplements based on plant enzymes are frequently prescribed together with vitamin B-12 and intrinsic-factor in the formula.

Part 3 – Reinoculate – This step includes the re-introduction of prebiotics and probiotics. This can be achieved with live bacteria supplements (probiotics). Prebiotics in the diet can support intestinal health, chiefly through the use of soluble fibre, such as soya.

Part 4 – Repair – Repair of the gut lining can become necessary as a result of candidiasis, leaky gut syndrome, long-term nutritional deficiencies, inflammation (colitis or Crohn's disease, for example), chronic infections and food allergies. The chief nutrients for promoting repair include L-glutamine, vitamin E, pantothenic acid/B-5), omega-3 and zinc.

Non-nutritional treatments for CFS

The Perrin technique

The Perrin technique has been developed by Dr Raymond Perrin, a registered osteopath and a specialist in treating CFS for more than 20 years. His researches have convinced him that CFS is a structural problem with diagnosable physical signs. The central theme of the technique is manual stimulation of the lymphatic system, in particular drainage from the brain and spinal cord to assist the health of the sympathetic nervous system. Dr Perrin believes that lymphatic drainage is the key to CFS symptoms and treatment. To quote his book, *The Perrin Technique – how to beat CFS/ME*: 'The Perrin technique stimulates the motion of fluid around the brain and spinal cord via cranial techniques. Treatment to the spine, as well as certain exercises, further aids drainage of these toxins out of the cerebrospinal fluid. Massage of the soft tissues in the head, neck, back and chest directs all the poisons out of the lymphatic system and into the blood, and eventually to the liver where they are broken down and readily detoxified.'

A similar technique known as the 'lymphatic pump' has been used by naturopathic osteopaths for over 50 years to stimulate lymphatic drainage. Dr Perrin's view is that there may be latent causes of CFS, sometimes for years before the actual CFS symptoms surface. These can include birth traumas, general traumas to the head and neck, developmental problems, including posture, and occupational or sporting injuries as a teenager. He suggests there may also be a genetic predisposition. He also believes that a 'toxic cocktail' can influence and overload the sympathetic nervous system (the part of the nervous system that controls the functioning of the body's internal organs), which can be further affected by other stress factors, including physical, allergic, emotional and infective influences. A final viral or bacterial trigger can produce the symptoms of CFS.

For any CFS patients who have had a history of head, neck or upper back traumas (such as whip-lash injuries), a consultation with a Perrin technique practitioner, or a practitioner who is familiar with lymphatic drainage, would be worthwhile. (Dr Perrin's book describing the technique is listed in Further reading. The list of useful names and addresses included in the book offers a comprehensive list of CFS/ME support groups.)

Pilates

Pilates has been described as a 'body conditioning regime'. It was founded by Joseph Pilates over 90 years ago. He was a German gymnast who original termed pilates 'contrology'. Pilates is an exercise-based system that aims to develop the body's 'centre' and achieve musculo-skeletal balance. This is done to create a stable core for all types of movement. The system serves to stretch, tone and mobilise the body with regular (often group) sessions.

Benefits of Pilates for CFS

The health benefits attributed to Pilates are many and varied, but in the context of relieving CFS symptoms the following benefits may be relevant:

1. Pilates emphasises the need for a correct breathing technique, to encourage flexibility of mind and body
2. Muscles are strengthened and made more flexible; this ensures increased joint flexibility

3. Pilates balances the body's muscles, conditioning and strengthening them for other sports and activities
4. Learning how to use the body in a more efficient way reduces muscle strain and fatigue; this is important for better posture and sports performance
5. Pilates encourages a feeling of accomplishment which assists confidence in other activities
6. A flexible spine is an important result of Pilates (such a requirement also being an essential component of the Perrin technique)
7. The absence of joint strain and fatigue is part of the Pilates method – many of the exercises are in the sitting or reclining position.

As stress – previous and current – plays a major part in causing CFS, a system like Pilates has a value in reducing the physical effects of stress. Although Pilates does not have a profound influence on our metabolism or chemistry, I have discussed its value with CFS patients who enjoy and benefit from regular classes. It may well be that group Pilates activity provides support and confidence to exhausted CFS and fibromyalgia patients. I believe it likely that Pilates, and other approaches to physical and mental balance (such as yoga, relaxation techniques, exercises), is more effective when practised within a group or class than in isolation at home.

Pilates has been described as 'dynamic yoga'. There are a few common concepts shared with Hatha yoga (see below).

Acupuncture

I trained as an acupuncturist for over three years in the late 1960s and I found it to be a safe, reliable and effective therapy for a large range of health conditions. However, although a patient's vitality can be increased with acupuncture, chiefly with the use of 'moxibustion' (applying heat), I usually found that the benefits were only transient.

The Chinese were not aware of the endocrine or the immune system when acupuncture was first used several thousand years ago, but we now know (see page 52) how important hormones, stress and immune-system efficiency are in the causation and treatment of CFS. Furthermore, the use of needles, massage and moxibustion in acupuncture is only a part of traditional

Chinese medicine. The system is based on the diagnosis and treatment of the body's energy (Chi). The therapies under the heading of Traditional Chinese Medicine include hydrotherapy, nutrition, plant therapy and massage, all in addition to acupuncture. It follows that the use of needles alone tends to have limitations. Acupuncture can provide a useful adjunct therapy when treating CFS, being of particular use in assisting relaxation, pain and other symptoms. Regrettably, I have never found it of lasting value when treating such conditions as iron-deficient anaemia, adrenal fatigue, hypothyroidism, candidiasis, mitochondrial failure, syndrome X or pernicious anaemia. Acupuncture has a value, but it is not a total treatment for CFS.

Hatha yoga

In keeping with many of the systems and disciplines covered in this section of the book, yoga has its value as a means of relieving stress. Yoga is one of the six orthodox systems of Hindu philosophy. In the West, the first four systems (the basis of Hatha yoga) have become widely popular as a method of encouraging relaxation and as a form of exercise. The breathing techniques and specific postures have been incorporated into many different fitness courses. Meditation is an important component of Hindu yoga, but not usually a part of Hatha yoga.

Hypnotherapy (hypnosis)

Franz Mesmer called hypnosis 'animal magnetism', which he made popular in the late 18th century with theatrical displays. The term hypnosis was coined by a British surgeon, James Braid, in the early part of the 19th century. The trance-like state induced by hypnosis has in fact been recognised in many cultures, reaching back to ancient times. Fortunately, the technique has left theatrical entertainments behind. It is currently used as hypnotherapy in dentistry, psychotherapy, obstetrics and generally to treat anxiety and depression, and to assist relaxation and pain control. Fatigued patients are often encouraged to learn self-hypnosis to achieve symptom-relief.

I have talked to patients who have experienced benefit from seeing a hypnotherapist, particularly in improving headaches, insomnia and the many symptoms resulting from previous and current stress. It is also of value in reducing reliance on drugs, alcohol and tobacco and can be prescribed to assist weight loss. Hypnosis is used to induce a state of relaxation in the patient; given the common symptoms seen in CFS of hyperventilation, agitation, insomnia and nervous exhaustion, its value is well established.

Patients in pain with the fibromyalgia syndrome (see page 57) can be helped to control, reduce or cope better with pain when using hypnotherapy.

Naturopathic treatment for CFS

Reduced cellular energy

Up to 90% of all our food needs to be converted into fuel. As I've described in earlier chapters, the currency of energy within our cells is adenosine triphosphate or 'ATP'. ATP is produced in the tiny biochemical factories that exist within each of our cells – the 'mitochondria', of which each cell in our body contains up to 3000. These tiny units produce the bulk of the energy our cells need. The process that produces this energy is known as 'cell respiration', which requires oxygen. The mitochondria also distribute the energy. As a result, many medical doctors and complementary practitioners consider that the reduction in performance, or failure, of the mitochondria is the chief cause of CFS.

When cellular energy is released, according to body need, the ATP in our cells is converted to adenosine diphosphate – 'ADP'. A complementary process – known as 'phosphorylation' – converts ADP back into vital ATP; this has been likened to a battery recharge, with the mitochondria being the rechargers and the ATP acting as the battery. So when the ATP (battery) 'runs down', becoming ADP, it needs to be recharged by the mitochondria. Figure 6.2 illustrates this energy cycle diagrammatically.

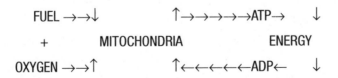

Figure 6.2: Energy production in our cells

Each mitochondrion maintains metabolic efficiency by supplying energy non-stop. This is to repair, heal, and deal with infections and inflammation in all the organs. It has been postulated that mitochondrial failure in excess of 70% of the total, can lead to a person's death. Although the human body consists of a huge variety of different cell types, in different tissues and organs, cellular energy production is identical in all cells and this is the same in all animals. Mitochondria are in fact the universal power units.

The concept of mitochondrial resuscitation is central to the successful treatment of CFS.

Testing for mitochondrial status

You may be wondering how mitochondrial malfunction is diagnosed and, more importantly for CFS patients, just how it is possible to treat low cellular energy. In chapter 5 (see page 119) I describe the tests that the Acumen laboratory provides for cellular energy (general) and ATP levels in cells (specific). Here I am concerned with the treatment of the deficiencies indicated by those tests, of which two typical examples are shown in Figures 6.3 and 6.4: Patient A is more or less normal; Patient B has CFS (see pages 170 to 173).

You should be aware that, although our energy production may appear simple within the cellular mitochondria, the biochemical background to this is in fact complex. There are therefore many ways in which that biochemical background can be adversely affected. If, as a result, the cyclical energy output slows and ATP levels within the mitochondria are depleted, fatigue will result, and potentially CFS. Reduction in mitochondrial activity, and injury to the mitochondria, can be caused by excessive exercise and overtraining. This chiefly occurs in endurance events (such as marathons), where overtraining to obtain top-level performances can cause what has been termed 'acquired mitochondrial myopathy'. This indicates that CFS does not always have a viral, nutritional or toxic cause.

Treatment for mitochondrial malfunction

Treatment for mitochondrial malfunction includes necessary life-style changes and specific therapeutic nutrients to assist energy production.

ATP (adenosine triphosphate), studies on neutrophils

ATP is hydrolysed to ADP and phosphate as the major energy source in muscle and other tissues. It is regenerated by oxidative phosphorylation of ADP in the mitochondria. When aerobic metabolism provides insufficient energy, extra ATP is generated during the anaerobic breakdown of glucose to lactic acid. ATP reactions require magnesium. ADP to ATP conversion can be blocked by environmental contaminants as can the translocator [TL] in the mitochondrial membrane. [TL] efficiency is also sensitive to pH and other metabolic-factor changes. [TL] defects may demand excessive ADP to AMP conversion (not re-converted to ADP or through to ATP). Defects in Mg-ATP, ADP – ATP conversion and enryme or [TL] blocking can all result in **chronic fatigue – a factor in any disease where biochemical energy availability is reduced.**

<u>**ATP**</u> whole cells:

With excess Mg added	**1.92** nmol/10^6 cells	1.6–2.9
(Standard method of measuring ATP)		
Endogenous Mg only	**1.15** nmol/10^6 cells	0.9–2.7
(Measured ATP result is lowered during intracellular magnesium deficiency)		
Ratio ATP/ATP^{Mg}	**0.6**	>0.65

<u>ADP to ATP conversion efficiency</u> (whole cells):

ATP^{Mg} (from above)	**1.92** nmol/10^6 cells	(1*)	1.6–2.9
ATP^{Mg} (inhibitor present)	**0.08** nmol/10^6 cells	(2*)	<0.3
ATP^{Mg} (inhibitor removed)	**1.37** nmol/10^6 cells	(3*)	>1.4
ADP to ATP efficiency [(3* − 2*0/(1* − 2*)] x 100 = **70.1%**		**>60**	
Blocking of active sites (2*/1*) x 100 = **4.2%**		**up to 14**	

<u>ADP-ATP TRANSLOCATOR</u> [TL] (mitochondria, not whole cells):

	ATP (pmol/10^6 cells)	Ref. range	change %	ref. range
Start	**366**	290–700		
[TL] '*out*'	**552**	410–950	**50.8**	over 35% (*Increase*)
				(in-vitro test) reflects ATP supply for cytoplasm
[TL] '*in*'	**140**	140–330	**58.3**	55 to 75% (*Decrease*)
				(in-vitro test) reflects normal use of ATP on energy demand

---

Comments   Rather low ATP-related magnesium: Otherwise-normal ATP profile.

Figure 6.3a: Typical 'normal' mitochondrial function profile

Chapter 6

Superoxide Dismutase Studies

A functional test looks at the in-vitro efficiency of the patient's red cell superoxide dismutase (SOD) when their neutrophil superoxide production is maximally stimulated. The activity of the individual forms of SOD are explored. General cell protection from damage by superoxide is provided by intracellular zinc:copper-SOD (Zn/Cu-SOD). Mitochondria are protected by manganese-dependent SOD (Mn-SOD). Extracellular SOD (EC-SOD – another Zn/Cu SODase) protects the nitric oxide pathways that relax vascular smooth muscle.

For each form of SODase, genetic variations are known, mutations can occur during excessive oxidative stress on DNA and polymorphisms can occur. DNA adducts can chemically block these genes.

Blood test results:

Test	Result	Units	Reference range
Functional test	38	%	Over 40 (mostly 41–47)
Zn/Cu-SOD	216	Enzyme activity (u)	240–410
Mn-SOD	142	Enzyme activity (u)	125–208
EC-SOD	44	Enzyme activity (u)	28–70

Gene studies:

SOD form	Gene(s)	Comments
Zn/Cu-SOD Coded on chromosome 21	Mild blocking (see DNA-adducts)	Low enzyme activity
Mn-SOD Coded on chromosome 6	Normal	Normal enzyme activity
EC-SOD Coded on chromosome 4	Normal	Normal enzyme activity

Figure 6.3b: Typical 'normal' mitochondrial function profile (cont'd)

ATP (adenosine triphosphate), studies on neutrophils

ATP is hydrolysed to ADP and phosphate as the major energy source in muscle and other tissues. It is regenerated by oxidative phosphorylation of ADP in the mitochondria. When aerobic metabolism provides insufficient energy, extra ATP is generated during the anaerobic breakdown of glucose to lactic acid. ATP reactions require magnesium. ADP to ATP conversion can be blocked by environmental contaminants as can the translocator [TL] in the mitochondrial membrane. [TL] efficiency is also sensitive to pH and other metabolic-factor changes. [TL] defects may demand excessive ADP to AMP conversion (not re-converted to ADP or through to ATP). Defects in Mg-ATP, ADP – ATP conversion and enryme or [TL] blocking can all result in **chronic fatigue – a factor in any disease where biochemical energy availability is reduced.**

__ATP__ whole cells:

With excess Mg added	**1.26** nmol/10^6 cells	1.6–2.9
(Standard method of measuring ATP)		
Endogenous Mg only	**0.67** nmol/10^6 cells	0.9–2.7
(Measured ATP result is lowered during intracellular magnesium deficiency)		
Ratio ATP/ATP^{Mg}	**0.53**	>0.65

__ADP to ATP conversion efficiency__ (whole cells):

ATP^{Mg} (from above)	**1.26** nmol/10^6 cells	(1*)	1.6–2.9
ATP^{Mg} (inhibitor present)	**0.34** nmol/10^6 cells	(2*)	<0.3
ATP^{Mg} (inhibitor removed)	**0.77** nmol/10^6 cells	(3*)	>1.4
ADP to ATP efficiency [(3* – 2*0/(1* – 2*)] x 100 = **46.7%**		**>60**	
Blocking of active sites (2*/1*) x 100 = **27%**		**up to 14**	

__ADP-ATP TRANSLOCATOR__ **[TL]** (mitochondria, not whole cells):

	ATP (pmol/10^6 cells)	**Ref. range**	**change %**	**ref. range**
Start	**218**	290–700		
[TL] 'out'	**271**	410–950	**24.3**	over 35% (*Increase*)
				(in-vitro test) reflects ATP supply for cytoplasm
[TL] 'in'	**174**	140–330	**20.2**	55 to 75% (*Decrease*)
				(in-vitro test) reflects normal use of ATP on energy demand

---

Comments	Very low whole-cell ATP	Low ATP-related magnesium
	27% blocking of active sites leading to:	Very poor ADP to ATP re-conversion
	Very low mt-ATP and very poor provision of ATP	
	Quite marked blocking of translocator function.	

Figure 6.4a: Typical mitochondrial function profile of a patient with chronic fatigue syndrome

<u>Superoxide Dismutase Studies</u>

A functional test looks at the in-vitro efficiency of the patient's red cell superoxide dismutase (SOD) when their neutrophil superoxide production is maximally stimulated. The activity of the individual forms of SOD are explored. General cell protection from damage by superoxide is provided by intracellular zinc:copper-SOD (Zn/Cu-SOD). Mitochondria are protected by manganese-dependent SOD (Mn-SOD). Extracellular SOD (EC-SOD – another Zn/Cu SODase) protects the nitric oxide pathways that relax vascular smooth muscle.

For each form of SODase, genetic variations are known, mutations can occur during excessive oxidative stress on DNA and polymorphisms can occur. DNA adducts can chemically block these genes.

Blood test results:

Test	Result	Units	Reference range
Functional test	33	%	Over 40 (mostly 41–47)
Zn/Cu-SOD	192	Enzyme activity (u)	240–410
Mn-SOD	138	Enzyme activity (u)	125–208
EC-SOD	22	Enzyme activity (u)	28–70

Gene studies:

SOD form	Gene(s)	Comments
Zn/Cu-SOD Coded on chromosome 21	Normal	Very low enzyme activity
Mn-SOD Coded on chromosome 6	Normal	Normal enzyme activity
EC-SOD Coded on chromosome 4	Normal	Low enzyme activity

Figure 6.4b: Typical mitochondrial function profile of a patient with chronic fatigue syndrome (cont'd)

Supplements

The following supplements may be prescribed, their selection and dosages being dependent on the results of the Acumen CFS profile (see page 119) and from the standard endocrine and biochemistry tests – for example, ferritin, vitamin B-12, red cell minerals, thyroid and adrenal status.

Co-enzyme Q-10

D-ribose

Intrinsic vitamin B-12

  (or B-12 injections)

L-carnitine

L-glutathione

Magnesium glycinate

N-acetyl-cysteine

NADH (vitamin B-3)

Omega-3 fatty acids

  (docosahexaenoic acid or DHA)

Super oxide dismutase

Vitamin B complex

Vitamin E

The Glossary at the end of the book describes these nutrients in more detail.

Cortisol – Cortisol is one of the two hormones measured using the adrenal stress profile (see page 121). Low cortisol levels may signify 'adrenal exhaustion'. Although the cause of stress usually needs to be treated, or if possible removed, specific adrenal glandular supplements can often improve the adrenal function within two to three months. Such a response can be seen in 'Elaine's story' on page 177. The specific glandular adrenal supplement that I prescribe provides 200 milligrams of adrenal concentrate with other nutrients that are involved in hormone balancing and regulation. When adrenal deficiency is diagnosed, medical doctors tend to prescribe adrenal hormone replacements (corticosteroids), the chief of which is prednisolone. This is a prescription-only drug and 5 milligrams of prednisolone delivers 20 milligrams of hydrocortisone (cortisol) (see the *British National Formulary* September 2011). You should be aware the hormone cortisone is converted to *cortisol*, but it is secreted in only minute amounts by the adrenal cortex. *Cortisol* is the major hormone of the adrenal cortex. Its pharmaceutical name is 'hydrocortisone'. *Prednisolone* is a synthetic hormone derived from cortisol. Those prescribing hydrocortisone do so with low 'physiological' dosages to avoid side-effects. However, naturopaths tend to rely on the glandular supplements which do not contain hormones and do not have side-effects.

DHEA (dehydroepiandrosterone) – DHEA is also measured using the adrenal stress profile. This is the only steroid hormone that I prescribe and only then when the adrenal test confirms a deficiency. It is completely free from side-effects and a single course of tablets over a six- to eight-week period is usually quite sufficient to normalise a patient's DHEA levels. The measures described can lead to improved ability to deal with stress and greater adrenal efficiency. The symptoms of stress, including anxiety and depression, may also need to be treated. This can often be achieved without recourse to anti-depressant drugs and the appropriately termed hypnotics and anxiolytic drugs. Medical doctors use these families of drugs to treat insomnia and anxiety, currently issuing 18 million prescriptions annually for these in the UK. They include the benzodiazepine group of drugs, which cause side-effects, drug dependency and severe withdrawal symptoms. The group includes Ativan (lorazepam) and Valium (diazepam) and 180-plus similar formulations. In contrast, naturopaths usually prescribe safer, non-addictive supplements to assist anxiety and insomnia. Many herbals have been used for centuries. These can include:

- Melatonin – A pineal gland hormone, used to treat jet-lag and to reset the sleep pattern and our biological clock
- 5HTP (5-hydroxytryptophan) – A plant-sourced tryptophan and a precursor to the neurotransmitter serotonin, which can itself be converted by the body to melatonin; 5HTP is also prescribed for anxiety. Tryptophan has been described by Dr Robert Atkins as, 'The best sleeping pill not on the market'
- Multi-minerals – A formula rich in calcium and magnesium can assist insomnia
- Vitamins – A strong B-complex is of value, as are high dosages of niacin (vitamin B-3) and pyridoxine (vitamin B-6)
- Herbs – Many different herbal remedies are prescribed to treat insomnia, and combination over-the-counter formulae are readily available. Herbs recommended include valerian, kava, hops, passionflower (passiflora), chamomile and skullcap.

GABA (gamma-amino butyric acid) – An amino acid that is also a neurotransmitter. Unlike its medical equivalent, which is valium, GABA is quite harmless, non-addictive and without withdrawal symptoms. It is chiefly prescribed as a tranquiliser, but it is useful for treating sleeplessness when stress is a component cause.

Essential life-style changes

With a diagnosis of mitochondrial failure or fatigue, the treatment programme may also need to include: treating stress and sleep disorders, dietary management, identifying possible food intolerances and allergies, reducing environmental stress and adopting an exercise routine.

Diet – A low-carbohydrate, low-sugar diet is preferred for treating fatigue. My low-carbohydrate diet is described earlier in this chapter (see page 149). Although food selection is obviously important, food quality is also a consideration. Locally produced, seasonal vegetables and sun-ripened fruit are best, having greater nutritional value that makes them more digestible. British shoppers are presented with all-season fruits and vegetables at their local supermarkets. Soft fruits, tomatoes, salad stuffs and many of the world's fruits and vegetable are available for 365 days each year.

Unfortunately, the commercial priority tends to favour appearance rather than flavour. I am fortunate to live in rural France. In the local weekly markets, the offering of fresh foods is based on when local produce becomes available. This means that asparagus, tomatoes, soft fruits, peas, beans, and even potatoes, have a seasonal 'window' when they can be purchased. Being locally produced and naturally ripened, they taste marvellous. The avoidance of processed food and choosing meat and fish on the basis of quality (where this can be afforded) should also be considered important.

Food allergies and intolerances – Testing for food allergies is yet another subject in medicine that is controversial. Testing is costly and often inconclusive. Food intolerances can lead to fatigue. If a patient suspects a food allergy, he/she can often describe a characteristic set of symptoms that usually tends to follow a typical age pattern and that preceded his/her current CFS. In childhood these tend to include histamine problems such as rhinitis, eczema, hives, asthma and catarrh. In adult life, typical symptoms include irritable bowel syndrome (IBS), migraines, indigestion with bloating, constipation and diarrhoea, and food allergies may be in addition to environmental allergies. There is frequently evidence of a family history, particularly with regard to lactose (milk sugar) intolerance and coeliac disease. **Lactose intolerance** arises from the absence of the lactose-digesting enzyme 'lactase', and is usually a problem from birth. **Coeliac disease** is a chronic malabsorption syndrome caused by intolerance to gluten, a protein found in wheat, oats, rye, barley, and other grains that are related to wheat. Many allergies and intolerances can cause a bewildering number of symptoms. CFS features in many of these groups, very often following years of misdiagnosis and treatment.

Mitochondrial failure – summary

The CFS profile blood tests, designed by Dr John McLaren-Howard at the Acumen laboratory in Devon, are the only tests available that can provide clues to the severity of a patient's CFS. As you know from earlier chapters, CFS can have many causes, and these causes are likely to be interrelated. As a result, should a patient's results to the Acumen test suggest mitochondrial fatigue, his/her treatment programme will probably need to be more comprehensive than a simple list of supplements. The first case-history, Elaine's story, outlines her treatment to illustrate this complexity. Life-style changes may be necessary, such as adequate sleep, stress control, paced exercises, improved diet and food allergy awareness, and underlying conditions may need to be treated be they blood deficiencies (iron, vitamin B-12, etc), hormonal insufficiencies (adrenal, thyroid etc), digestive conditions (candidiasis, leaky gut, etc), blood sugar problems, suspected allergies, poor immune system function, or poor liver status. Obviously, testing for these problems goes well beyond the scope of a patient's DIY capabilities. It seems an obvious first step therefore to identify and, where possible, improve life-style problems that may contribute to CFS.

Elaine's story

Elaine was a 38-year-old, single, self-employed woman who had suffered severe, chronic fatigue for eight years when she first consulted me. She described a catalogue of other symptoms aside from the fatigue. These included muscle and joint pain with stiffness, this being worse on rising, severe anxiety and concentration problems, mood swings and repeated infections. Elaine was also overweight by 3 stone (42 pounds or 19 kilograms).

Her GP had decided that her symptoms were chiefly a result of stress related to her work, Elaine being the CEO of her own company. This diagnosis had been endorsed by the complete absence of any significant results from the blood tests her doctor had requested. The treatment subsequently prescribed by her GP consisted of anti-depressants and anti-inflammatory drugs, which Elaine had declined to take.

When in her late 20s, Elaine had been given a diagnosis of mild hypothyroidism, the cause of which was again thought to be stress. This was 'cured' with a short course of low-dosage thyroxine. At this time, she was also prone to experimenting with various 'leisure drugs', in particularly Ecstasy, in addition to which she relied on frequent coffees, alcohol, and a high-sugar diet to provide much needed, but temporary, energy.

With the onset of her severe fatigue and muscle pain, she had made the wise decision to improve her diet and aim for a healthier life-style. Although she had experienced some symptom relief, it was minimal.

When she consulted me, her fatigue, pain and anxiety persisted, on a daily basis.

I requested a batch of tests that can often provide useful clues with fibromyalgia-type symptoms and chronic fatigue. This blood test profile, known as the 'fatigue profile', included tests for ferritin (iron reserves), vitamin B-12 and her thyroid profile (free T4, T3 and TSH). I also requested an adrenal stress profile. This saliva test measures the adrenal hormones cortisol and dehydroepiandrosterone (DHEA) and is a valuable indicator of the effects of past and current stress. Elaine's Acumen results are shown in Figure 6.5 (see page 179).

Elaine's blood test showed borderline anaemia, a low vitamin B-12 level and a low to normal thyroid output. Moreover the adrenal test confirmed very low levels of cortisol and DHEA. Extreme results such as hers are usually defined as 'adrenal exhaustion'. Such an adrenal status is usually a result of long-term stress, coupled with an unhealthy diet and life-style. Not surprisingly, poor ability to deal with stress is a common feature. Unfortunately, as with Elaine,

ATP (adenosine triphosphate), studies on neutrophils

ATP is hydrolysed to ADP and phosphate as the major energy source in muscle and other tissues. It is regenerated by oxidative phosphorylation of ADP in the mitochondria. When aerobic metabolism provides insufficient energy, extra ATP is generated during the anaerobic breakdown of glucose to lactic acid. ATP reactions require magnesium. ADP to ATP conversion can be blocked by environmental contaminants as can the translocator [TL] in the mitochondrial membrane. [TL] efficiency is also sensitive to pH and other metabolic-factor changes. [TL] defects may demand excessive ADP to AMP conversion (not re-converted to ADP or through to ATP). Defects in Mg-ATP, ADP – ATP conversion and enryme or [TL] blocking can all result in **chronic fatigue – a factor in any disease where biochemical energy availability is reduced.**

ATP whole cells:

With excess Mg added	**1.43** nmol/10^6 cells	1.6–2.9
(Standard method of measuring ATP)		
Endogenous Mg only	**0.87** nmol/10^6 cells	0.9–2.7
(Measured ATP result is lowered during intracellular magnesium deficiency)		
Ratio ATP/ATP^{Mg}	**0.61**	>0.65

ADP to ATP conversion efficiency (whole cells):

ATP^{Mg} (from above)	**1.43** nmol/10^6 cells	(1*)	1.6–2.9
ATP^{Mg} (inhibitor present)	**0.08** nmol/10^6 cells	(2*)	<0.3
ATP^{Mg} (inhibitor removed)	**0.78** nmol/10^6 cells	(3*)	>1.4
ADP to ATP efficiency [(3* – 2*0/(1* – 2*)] x 100 = **51.9%**		**>60**	
Blocking of active sites (2*/1*) x 100 = **5.6%**		**up to 14**	

ADP-ATP TRANSLOCATOR [TL] (mitochondria, not whole cells):

	ATP (pmol/10^6 cells)	Ref. range	change %	ref. range
Start	**252**	290–700		
[TL] 'out'	**320**	410–950	**26.9**	over 35% (*Increase*)
				(in-vitro test) reflects ATP supply for cytoplasm
[TL] 'in'	**48**	140–330	**80.9**	55 to 75% (*Decrease*)
				(in-vitro test) reflects normal use of ATP on energy demand

Comments	Very low whole-cell ATP	Low ATP-related magnesium
	No significant blocking of active sites	Poor ADP to ATP re-conversion
	Very low mt-ATP and very poor provision of 'new' mt-ATP	
	Rapid depletion of ATP on increased energy demand.	

Figure 6.5: Elaine's mitochondrial function profile

the symptoms of adrenal exhaustion can themselves become an additional cause of stress, leading to a vicious circle. This is so often a feature of CFS and fibromyalgia that the naturopathic concept of treating the causes of the disease and not the symptoms may need to be amended to include, 'But also provide symptom relief where possible' – in order to resolve the 'vicious circle' that is so often part of the adrenal fatigue or exhaustion syndrome.

I requested one further test for Elaine – the ATP fatigue profile (see Fig 6.5, page 179). The test results showed that energy conversion in her cells was poor, with rapid depletion of ATP (adenosine triphosphate) with any increased energy demand. The results also confirmed a low whole-cell ATP level. Such results are all consistent with a diagnosis of CFS-linked fibromyalgia.

Elaine's treatment plan

With her morning lethargy, adrenal depletion and anxiety, coupled with her sugar-rich diet, Elaine was almost certainly a candidate for frequent episodes of low blood sugar. I therefore advised her to follow a low-carbohydrate, frequent-meal diet, known as an 'LBS maintenance diet' (see below, page 181). I also prescribed my Glucose Tolerance Factor Complex™ that I formulated for Nutri Advanced 10 years ago. This complex contains many nutrients that are involved in balancing our blood glucose levels, including chromium, B-complex vitamins, magnesium, potassium, adrenal glandular concentrate and zinc. Elaine's weight problem could also eventually be reduced by following such a diet.

The Acumen ATP test had also clearly shown that Elaine suffered from problems with energy production and recycling at cellular level – that is, mitochondrial failure, resulting in poor ATP production. Oxygen within our cells can be damaging unless the mitochondria contain anti-oxidants. These include co-enzyme Q-10, lipoic acid and L-carnitine. After I had analysed the results of Elaine's tests it was clear to me that her energy production at cell level was impaired. Her metabolic rate was severely depressed, this being reflected in her low adrenal and thyroid activity and many of her symptoms. Under-functioning adrenal glands are prone to cause muscle pain and stiffness (the adrenal steroids are our natural painkillers), low blood sugar levels (particularly after the night fast) and reduced immune efficiency. Elaine's borderline iron-deficient anaemia and her low blood level of vitamin B-12 were also contributing to her many symptoms, particularly her very low stamina.

Elaine's supplement programme

To provide antioxidants, essential nutrients and glandular support I prescribed the following supplement programme for Elaine: L-carnitine, intrinsic B-12, co-enzyme Q-10, magnesium glycinate, NADH (vitamin B-3), Nutri Thyroid (Glandular), Thyro Complex, Nutri Adrenal Extra (Glandular) Hemagenics (iron), GTF complex, D-ribose (specialised sugar) and omega-3 (fish oil capsules). The Thyro Complex and the GTF Complex both contain multi-nutrients as 'back-up' support (zinc, B-complex, vitamins C and E, etc).

Elaine's maintenance diet for low blood sugar

I recommended Elaine follow my 'maintenance diet for low blood sugar':

Breakfast – The ideal breakfast is a wholegrain cereal or 1 slice of wholemeal bread and sugar-free jam or marmalade plus fresh fruit. Sugar-free muesli can be purchased or homemade. For additional protein use sugar-free soya milk on the cereal; this is more palatable when diluted 25% with water or fruit juice. If appetite allows, select from the following: egg (scrambled, poached, boiled or omelette), low-sugar baked beans, sugar-free ham or grilled lean bacon, cheese on toast, sardines on toast, grilled or steamed fish with 1 slice of wholemeal bread (may be toasted) or brown rice, roll and butter or soya margarine as desired.

Lunch – Meat, fish, cheese or eggs, salad (large serving of lettuce, tomato, etc, with French dressing or mayonnaise), vegetables if desired. Only one slice of wholemeal bread, toast or crispbread with butter or soya margarine. For dessert – cheese, yoghurt or fruit. Beverage (see Notes).

Dinner – Soup if desired, vegetables or salad, liberal portion of meat, fish or poultry. Only one slice of wholemeal bread if desired. For dessert – cheese, yoghurt or one piece of fruit. Beverage (see Notes).
NB – Dinner and lunch may be reversed.

Supper (as late as possible) – Crispbread with pâté, cheese, ham or cold meat with butter. Beverage (see below) or milk. Natural yoghurt.

Notes

- Drink raw milk if available.
- Avoid wherever possible the use of sugar substitutes. 'Sugar-free' soft drinks should be used very cautiously.
- Fruit and vegetables – Avoid excess dates, raisins and bananas as they have a high sugar content
- Beverages – Any natural coffee substitutes or decaffeinated coffee; herb teas or weak China or Indian tea
- Alcohol – If acceptable, limit to one glass of dry white wine with the dinner.
- Tobacco – To be avoided, as should smoky atmospheres whenever possible.
- Avoid all products containing sugar (such as glucose, fructose, sucrose, dextrose, syrup, molasses and honey).
- When using cereal, bread rice or pasta, obtain good-quality, naturally produced wholemeal or wholegrain products.
- On special occasions the use of diabetic ice-cream, chocolates and sweets could be considered in small amounts.

NB: This diet should be used only when under direct supervision of a practitioner.

Elaine's response to treatment

Elaine's symptoms improved slowly. Her initial response to the diet changes was not good, as she suffered stomach wind and heartburn. However, she stuck to it and after three months her vitality began to improve and she noticed she had more energy on rising. After four months her concentration also began to improve. Nevertheless, her long-term anxiety had not really changed so I prescribed a course of GABA (gamma-amino butyric acid). This is a safe nutritional tranquiliser, sometimes referred to as 'nature's valium'. It is an amino acid (protein) and a neurotransmitter. The body converts glutmate to GABA, with vitamin B-6 (pyridoxine) being essential for this conversion. GABA is of particular value for treating anxiety, insomnia and depression.

After six months of treatment Elaine was able to reduce her supplements to a maintenance dosage. Subsequent tests of her cellular energy, adrenal function and anaemia status showed reassuringly that these had improved in line with the progress in her symptoms.

Iron-deficient anaemia (IDA)

When mild iron-deficient anaemia is diagnosed, a diet emphasising iron-rich foods can provide sufficient treatment to remedy the deficiency. Such a diet needs to be coupled with the avoidance of nutrients that are known to inhibit iron absorption.

Iron-rich foods and drinks

I recommend the following iron-rich foods:

> Liver – calves' liver is the best source
> Red meats, in particular offal meats
> Fish, in particular shellfish
> Egg yolks
> Dark green vegetables and salads
> Dried fruit – apricots, raisins, figs, dates, prunes
> Cherries and berries generally
> Bananas
> Grapes
> Legumes
> Whole grains
> Black cherry juice
> Red wine (up to two glasses daily).

Iron supplements

Iron supplements are best taken separately from food – that is, 30 minutes before or 60 minutes after meals. The following foods and drinks should be reduced or avoided as they tend to inhibit iron absorption: tea, coffee, alcohol and calcium-rich foods (such as milk, cheese and cream). It has been shown that women, in particular, are able to absorb 50% more iron from a meal that has a low calcium content.

Vitamin C taken with iron supplements can assist absorption, the recommended dosage being 400–500 milligrams of vitamin C with each iron source. Should iron supplements cause digestive symptoms – which can include nausea, heartburn, constipation and diarrhoea – liquid supplements may be appropriate, providing a more comfortable option.

Iron can also be delivered by intra-muscular injection, or by infusions, directly into the blood. When prescribing iron supplements for anaemic patents, I usually recommend the Nutri Advanced product Hemagenics, this being a synergistic (it contains a number of ingredients that work together), bio-available (easily absorbed) source of iron as it uses a highly absorbable form of iron, iron bisglycinate. Iron unfortunately competes with the minerals copper and zinc at absorption sites in the intestines. This explains the very poor absorption of the commonly prescribed ferrous sulphate and many other iron salts. (Only around 8–10% is absorbed.) Furthermore, the actual iron content of ferrous sulphate at 300 milligrams strength is only 60 milligrams. Each tablet of Hemagenics contains:

Vitamins B-1, B-6, B-12	Iron (as iron bisglycinate)
Calcium	Copper
Folate	Succinic acid
Phosphorus	Glycine.

Iron-deficient anaemia – summary

Iron-deficient anaemia (IDA) is the commonest cause of fatigue. It should therefore always be prioritised as the 'first step' in the diagnosis and treatment of CFS. The level of blood ferritin is the best indicator of our iron status.

An iron-rich diet is important for treatment, coupled with appropriate iron supplements. However, such measures may prove to be of only transient help unless the cause is also addressed. The most frequently seen causes usually involve blood-loss, such as from excessively heavy periods. Serious underlying causes of blood loss, such as cancer, stomach ulcer and intestinal disease, may need to be excluded before commencing treatment.

As described in chapter 5 (Diagnosis), the usual anaemia profile that is obtained by a GP or a hospital can often not include the all-important ferritin test. I have seen many patients with normal blood haemoglobin and normal iron, but with very low ferritin, indicating IDA. Exhausted patients are advised to request a copy of any anaemia tests and double check that ferritin has been included. It is worth remembering that the ferritin test (iron stores) is seen as the best test for determining a patient's iron status.

Liz's story

Liz was a 42-year-old single mother who had been experiencing chronic fatigue for two years when she first consulted me. With two children aged eight and six years, and with three student lodgers, she was under considerable stress, with a heavy workload. She also worked full-time as a medical secretary. Unfortunately, her GP considered that Liz's fatigue was a result of stress from her workload and an impending divorce. In spite of this diagnosis, her GP requested blood tests, which revealed the following results (with 'N/R' signifying 'normal range'):

Ferritin (iron stores)   17.8 µg/l (N/R 12–300)
Haemoglobin   13.3 g/dl (N/R 11.5–15.5)

As these results were within the normal ranges used by the laboratory, no treatment was offered, except anti-depressants.

Ferritin

Ferritin has been described as the most sensitive and reliable non-invasive test for detecting iron-deficient anaemia (IDA), sometimes referred to as the 'stamina factor'. Ferritin (iron stores) can become depleted in IDA before the haemoglobin (blood iron). While the NHS 'normal range' for ferritin is a very low 12 to 300 micrograms per litre, private laboratories recommend a range of 30 or 40 to 150, and many practitioners and laboratory workers consider that 40 is the lowest acceptable level. I therefore considered Liz's ferritin level at 17.8 to be too low.

Not surprisingly, Liz had other health problems, including adrenal fatigue with resulting episodes of low blood sugar. She also experienced heavy periods which contributed to her low ferritin. I recommended that she follow my iron-rich diet coupled with the Hemagenics supplement and vitamin C (to take with each dosage). Her GP co-operated by prescribing combined oral contraception to provide Liz with a three- to four-month respite from her periods and agreed to refer her to see a consultant to find the cause of her excessively heavy periods.

An adrenal stress profile saliva test had confirmed a state of adrenal fatigue with low cortisol levels. I therefore recommended that Liz should also take an adrenal glandular supplement (Nutri Adrenal Extra), another Nutri Advanced product that, although being hormone-free, can within three to four months greatly improve adrenal efficiency. (All glandulars from Nutri Advanced are sourced from New Zealand cows. In my experience they are free from side-effects. Unlike steroid hormones, they do not create dependency.)

With her supplement programme taking effect, the absence of periods and an appointment pending to see a gynaecologist, Liz began to feel more vital and more relaxed.

After four months of treatment, I requested a repeat ferritin test and another adrenal stress profile. This showed her cortisol status had improved by 30% and her ferritin level had increased from her original 17.8 µg/l to 38. More improvement was needed, but Liz was beginning to break the vicious circle that her ill-health had developed into. Her exhaustion had exacerbated her poor stress handling, which had added in turn to her exhaustion. It was clear that IDA was not the sole cause of Liz's fatigue, but resolving her low ferritin level was a necessary first step to improving her fatigue and other symptoms.

Vitamin B-12 deficiency

Many people, if asked, would state that vitamin B-12 deficiency is caused by pernicious anaemia. There are in fact more common causes of vitamin B-12 deficiency and pernicious anaemia is only one of the causes.

Our body needs 13 vitamins, and vitamin B-12 is the only vitamin that we cannot obtain from plants, or sunlight. To obtain vitamin B-12 we need to eat poultry, meat, eggs, fish or dairy products. Unfortunately, there is evidence that the majority of B-12 deficient patients eat plenty of B-12 rich foods. (It is only vegans who need to take regular supplements of B-12.) The problem is that their body cannot sufficiently absorb it. As described in earlier chapters, this may be the result of:

- Pernicious anaemia (the absence of 'instrinsic factor' in the stomach, without which B-12 cannot be absorbed – see page 113)
- Reduced stomach acid (generally in the elderly) due to atrophic

gastritis or achlorhydria; stomach acid is required to separate vitamin B-12 from protein

- Drugs that compromise vitamin B-12 absorption, including proton pump inhibitors (eg Omeprazole), biguanides used to treat diabetes (eg Metformin), potassium supplements (eg Slow-K), H-2 blockers (eg Tagamet), and a large family of ant-acid drugs
- Nitrous oxide anaesthetics
- Excessive alcohol
- Mercury amalgam.

Treatment for vitamin B-12 deficiency

The current prescription for B-12 deficiency in the UK is a 1 millilitre injection of 1 mg/ml (milligrams per millilitre) hydroxocobalamin, every three months. Unfortunately, vitamin B-12 being water-soluble, the vitamin will largely disappear in the recipient's urine. This has produced a situation within the NHS, where the most contentious issue that concerns those with pernicious anaemia is that of injection frequency.

Twenty years ago, I was able to obtain a Swiss vitamin B-12 injectable called Nova B-douze. This was 10 mg/ml B-12 in strength in a 2 millilitre phial. The B-12 was in the form known as cyancobalamine. At that time I was working at the Basingstoke Clinic and, with a group of naturopaths and osteopaths, regularly treating CFS patients, but also people with neuralgia, sciatica, referred pain, post-herpetic neuralgia (pain after shingles) and many other conditions, all of which benefited from vitamin B-12 injections. We usually gave such patients three to four Nova B-douze intramuscular injections weekly, that being 30 milligrams per week.

It is now impossible to obtain any similar dosages from French pharmacists in excess of 1 mg/2 ml. Fortunately, the very small disposable syringes that I provide for my patients mean that they can very easily inject vitamin B-12 on a daily basis. As a back-up treatment, I usually provide the Nutri Advanced Intrinsi B12/Folate™ tablets, each of which provides 500 micrograms of B-12, 800 micrograms folate, plus the intrinsic factor (20 micrograms) to facilitate absorption.

It has been shown that oral doses of vitamin B-12 in excess of 2000 micrograms can, in some patients, replace injections. Such a dosage would be quite easy with the Intrinsi formula, with four tablets daily. However, a typical B-complex may only contain 25–50 micrograms of B-12 per tablet – that makes for a lot of tablets!

Many practitioners, with the knowledge that vitamin B-12 injections are inexpensive, safe and virtually painless, tend to opt for the injections for their patients in preference to an oral source.

Michael's story

Michael was a solicitor aged 58 years when he first consulted me. Although he complained of eight to 10 symptoms his main concern was his progressively debilitating fatigue. He was tired on waking and his poor physical and mental energy had both got worse over a period of two-and-a-half to three years. So much so, that he had been obliged to reduce his workload in his legal practice, where he was a senior partner. He considered that he had become noticeably 'clumsy and forgetful' and he felt that solicitors should not be forgetful.

Michael had been subject to a great deal of stress over the previous eight years, beginning with a very unpleasant divorce, which was the chief cause of a subsequent stomach ulcer coupled with a stomach tumour. After six years of regular vomiting and nausea (which his GP diagnosed as migraine) and frequent ant-acid drug use, he was finally advised to have a partial gastrectomy. A large percentage of his stomach was surgically removed. Michael's fatigue worsened after the surgery. Although it is well known that vitamin B-12 deficiency can result from stomach surgery, his blood vitamin B-12 was not checked.

In common with many blood tests that are requested to identify possible deficiencies (such as iron, hypothyroidism), blood B-12 levels do not always conveniently match a patient's symptoms. Michael's blood B-12 was within the UK 'normal range', but at the lower end of the range. As I describe in chapter 5 on Diagnosis (see page 112), the European normal range for blood B-12 is significantly lower than the ranges used in the USA. In the USA, Michael's results would have been graded very definitely as 'too low'. This, coupled with his symptoms (debilitating and worsening fatigue, clumsiness, forgetfulness) confirmed deficiency.

Although Michael had other health problems, I decided to give his B-12 deficiency priority treatment and commenced a course of vitamin B-12 intramuscular injections twice weekly for one month. I also prescribed a vitamin B-12 tablet that included the intrinsic factor and folic acid in the formula, for enhanced absorption.

When patients present several disorders requiring treatment, it is very tempting to treat the symptoms all at once for rapid and maximum relief. However, there is a value in treating their problems in sequence. Such a schedule can enable me to assess the impact of each health condition on a person's symptom picture. With Michael's fatigue, he began to experience noticeable relief after four weeks of vitamin B-12 treatment. He also had problems with his diet, being overweight, and his poor stress-handling over many years had caused adrenal fatigue. This was to require six to nine months of adrenal glandular supplements before resolving, but with the B-12 injections he made a good start and his CFS began to improve.

Michael is typical of many fatigued patients who consult me. The pattern of his symptoms related to at least four areas of ill-health that all required accurate diagnosis and effective treatment. When I discuss fatigued patients with other naturopaths and medical doctors, there is general agreement that fatigue with a single cause is very rare.

Low thyroid (hypothyroidism)

I have described hypothyroidism and the obstacles to diagnosing it, at least in the UK, in chapter 5 on diagnosis (see pages 102–104). There are also problems with the standard approach to treatment offered by the NHS in the UK, which I will review before describing the naturopathic approach.

The standard medical treatment for an underactive thyroid consists of replacement thyroid hormones – thyroxine (T4) or triiothyronine (T3). (T3 is very rarely prescribed in the UK except as an intravenous injection to treat hypothyroid comas.) T4 is converted into T3 by cells in the liver and kidneys. Around 80% of our T3 in circulation is produced in this way. The thyroid gland itself produces the remaining 20% of T3.

Many practitioners consider that blood tests are not a satisfactory method of assessing thyroid efficiency. They prefer to assess the patient's symptom severity. They point to the variations between different laboratories in so-called 'normal ranges' for the thyroid hormones. In his excellent book *Recovering with T3*, Paul Robinson sums this up with the following comment: 'Ranges are actually statistical concepts that cannot be used as absolute cast-in-stone diagnostic or therapeutic ranges.'

Unfortunately, the role of a patient's iron status (ferritin), and the possibility of adrenal malfunction, rarely feature as part of the hypothyroid syndrome in western medicine. I frequently see CFS hypothyroid patients who are taking prescribed thyroxine yet claim there is no improvement in their symptoms. In common with many naturopaths and other non-medical practitioners, I prescribe glandular supplements for my hypothyroid patients. Unlike replacement hormones (such as thyroxine), the glandulars support the thyroid with 'organ specific', non-hormonal substances. My preference is for New Zealand bovine (BSE-free) glands, which serve to support the function of the human thyroid. The notion of 'like cures like' is a very old concept. Supplementation with thyroid tissue concentrates can provide safe and effective thyroid support.

In addition to thyroid glandulars, I also regularly prescribe the supplement Thyro Complex™. I designed this formula for the Nutri Advanced company some years ago, to deliver nutrients to the thyroid gland. It is used to provide support for those on thyroid glandulars and also those patients on thyroxine. Thyro Complex contains the following nutrients and herbs:

Magnesium	Zinc
Vitamin C	Vitamins B-1, B-2, B-3 and B-6
L-tyrosine	Manganese
Calcium	Selenium
Vitamin E	Liquorice root
L-carnitine	Copper
DL-phenylalanine	Vitamin A
Iodine	Folic acid.

With thyroxine treatment of over 100 micrograms daily, a dependency can develop as the patient's own thyroid can become less efficient. In the UK, the prescription for thyroxine is classed as a 'free prescription', in common with insulin and certain drugs. This is because the prescriptions are usually for life. Because the thyroxine usually fails to improve the patient's actual thyroid health, its use cannot be discontinued. This is quite different from the thyroid glandular treatment. Any improvement in test results and symptoms is a result of the patient's own thyroid gland increasing in efficiency. When a normal level of T4 is achieved, coupled with corresponding symptom-relief, I quite often advise patients to discontinue the supplements. With chronic, long-term or elderly patients I may recommend a lower dosage maintenance programme. This is usually backed up with an annual review, which includes blood tests.

Low thyroid – summary

Hypothyroidism is a frequently seen cause of chronic fatigue. It may also be a symptom of other health problems. These include iron-deficient anaemia (IDA) and adrenal insufficiency. Although the thyroid gland can influence our metabolism it can also reflect our metabolism, particularly with chronic infections and stress. Simply 'topping up' a CFS patient's blood thyroxine may not provide a complete solution.

Mary's story

I am including Mary's case history as she showed typical symptoms of hypothyroidism, yet her blood tests had returned 'normal' and her dosage of thyroxine had remained the same for 12 years. When she first consulted me, Mary was a 55-year-old secretary. She was at least 2 stone (28 pounds or 12.7 kilos) overweight and suffered from hair loss, poor skin quality, cold extremities and both physical and mental fatigue. She was depressed and increasingly concerned over her poor short-term memory and concentration. Her libido was non-existent and she suffered from insomnia.

At my request Mary obtained copies of the results of blood tests her GP had requested over the previous eight years; the testing had been done approximately twice annually. A typical NHS cost-cutting exercise is for laboratory technicians to refuse to test free T4 levels if the level for thyroid stimulating hormone (TSH) is 'normal'. I have spoken to GPs who have expressed annoyance and frustration that the free T4 has been crossed off their blood test request forms. As I discussed in chapter 5 (see pages 102 to 104), TSH is not even a thyroid hormone. It does not always reflect mild or borderline hypothyroid states, even when free T4 is below the normal range.

Mary's test results showed her TSH levels to be normal. Her last free T4 test results were from three years earlier, and those were also 'normal'. Her GP was therefore reassured (wrongly) that Mary's thyroid was working without fault and her thyroxine dosage was appropriate.

This commonly seen scenario serves to demonstrate yet another defect in modern thyroid testing. The normal ranges for free T4 test results in European laboratories do not distinguish between patients taking thyroxine and patients not taking thyroxine. As the test involves measuring a hormone that patients may be taking each day, it seems logical to allow for the thyroxine dosage when defining the normal range. In America it is quite usual to offer two normal ranges – a range for those people who are not taking thyroxine and a higher normal range for those who are taking thyroxine (with some allowance for dosage). I have seen test results for American patients who are taking thyroxine and these are usually qualified with the comment, 'As this patient is on...dosage of thyroxine, her normal range should be...'

Mary did not have a recent free T4 test result available and the interpretation of all her previous results had been based on a 'normal range' far too low for her prescribed thyroxine dosage. This resulted in a situation I see all too often – a fatigued patient who had been reassured that all was well.

I prescribed nutritional and thyroid glandular supplements and her symptoms responded well. Within four months her free T4 blood test results had increased by 20%.

Although I advised Mary to continue with her current dosage of thyroxine, I have in the past often recommended patients to reduce or even to discontinue their prescribed thyroxine, but only after ensuring that their blood test results and symptom picture had normalised. I have no objection to hormone-replacement therapy (such as in type I diabetes, where insulin can be essential), but when a patient is improved in general health through changes in diet and selected supplement use, it is sometimes possible to enjoy better health without supplementary hormones.

Adrenal fatigue

Adrenal fatigue, or insufficiency, is a common feature of CFS. I find approximately 80% of my CFS patients have this problem; the good news is it can be diagnosed and treated.

The current diagnosis and treatment of adrenal fatigue in mainstream medicine demonstrate the shortcomings in CFS diagnosis. I frequently discuss the value of adrenal gland function with my fatigued patients, in particular the role of the hormones cortisol and DHEA. Cortisol, which is made from cholesterol, is seen as our stress-handling hormone. In fact it has other vital functions including immune support, blood sugar control, thyroid support, energy production and blood pressure control. Lack of cortisol can cause exhaustion, depression, low blood pressure and weight loss. A very low level of cortisol is known as Addison's disease; this is dangerous and can result in death, usually from kidney failure or shock (adrenal crisis). Addison's is usually seen as an auto-immune condition. A level of cortisol that is too high is known as Cushing's syndrome.

Some of my patients have been reassured by their GPs that their adrenals are normal as the tests requested to identify adrenal problems have come back negative. The test used for suspected Addison's disease, or severe 'hypoadrenalism', is the 'short Synacthen test' (SST). This test does not measure adrenal insufficiency capacity, only adrenal collapse. It is a typical 'black or white' routine, so often seen in medical diagnosis. Functional 'shades of grey' are discounted and simply not recognised. The term 'adrenal fatigue' is used to describe adrenal inefficiency but not severe deficiency. It is sometimes referred to as adrenal exhaustion or collapse. Many CFS patients have under-functioning adrenals with low cortisol and DHEA levels. They do *not* have Addison's disease.

Private medical practitioners, who treat CFS, will usually prescribe hydrocortisone for adrenal fatigue, or the synthetic derivative named prednisolone. Naturopaths will prescribe nutritional adrenal support and probably adrenal glandular supplements. Low DHEA levels can be quickly corrected by taking DHEA, this being a very safe steroid hormone, which I supply for my patients; a three-month course is often quite sufficient.

The test of choice to diagnose adrenal fatigue is the adrenal stress profile, this being a saliva test, done at home, that involves four samples to measure cortisol status and two samples to measure DHEA over a 12-hour period. The all-important 'total daily cortisol' is noted, as is the DHEA/cortisol ratio.

This valuable test provides precise information on a patient's stress load and stress handling, but it also serves as a guide to specific supplement dosage requirements and gives some idea of the treatment time-scale. Repeat tests, approximately every three months, provide a useful indication of progress and serve to offer clues when compared with previous results.

Testing hormones in the saliva is seen by many practitioners as being preferable to blood and urine tests as it identifies 'shades of grey' in the way blood tests cannot. The only hormones for which a reliable saliva test kit has yet to be designed are the thyroid hormones.

The test procedure is very simple. I contact Genova Diagnostics, based in New Malden, Surrey, who post an adrenal stress profile kit to the patient. Everything needed is included. The saliva samples are posted by the patient to Genova, after freezing them over night. Preparation is simple; I usually recommend that Sunday is the best testing day to avoid any weekend postal delays. I am often asked by patients doing the test, 'Do I have to relax on the test day?' I am able to reassure them that it can be a 'normal' day for them.

Test results tend to reflect the effects of long-term stress, often over a period of months or even years, if the stress is ongoing. This very useful test cost around £80 and my patents usually see the results as good value for money.

To indicate the value of the adrenal stress test for assessing the effects of treatment I have included below a set of before and after results. The increase in cortisol output matched the improvement in this patient's symptoms in a very satisfactory manner. She has been discharged since, but I have recommended an annual adrenal test as a check up.

Mrs X – Typical adrenal stress profile results

Mrs X, a 62-year-old widow, had suffered from the following symptoms for over four years when she came to see me: chronic fatigue, episodes of low blood sugar, frequent palpitations, 'always cold', widespread muscle and joint pain and stiffness, anxiety and depression. She had experienced a great deal of stress with her husband's sudden death five years earlier and a hysterectomy four years before.

In the absence of any other obvious health problem, I reckoned that Mrs X was suffering from the very typical symptoms of adrenal exhaustion. Her blood testing showed mild, borderline hypothyroidism. Nonetheless her fatigue, worse on rising with energy slumps if meals were delayed, and her muscle and joint pain, all pointed to adrenal insufficiency with resulting low blood sugar. Consequently, the adrenal stress test seemed an appropriate first step in her diagnosis. This confirmed a diagnosis of adrenal fatigue and showed a very low 'total daily cortisol'. The test results from the five tests that Mrs X had over a 20-month period are shown below. Fortunately, the improvements in these figures matched almost exactly the changes in her general health, with subsequent reduction in muscle and joint pain, greater vitality and a more optimistic and calmer state of mind. (I have not included her DHEA levels as these were within the normal reference ranges in all the tests.)

1st Test
Every one of the four cortisol samples gave a result that was below the reference limits
Total daily cortisol – 7.3 nmol/l   (Range 21–41)

2nd Test   (4 months later)
Again, all but one of the four cortisol samples was still below the reference limits
Total daily cortisol – 10.9 nmol/l   (Range 21–41)

3rd Test   (8 months later)
Two of the cortisol samples were still below the reference limits
Total daily cortisol – 13.3 nmol/l   (Range 21–41)

4th Test   (14 months after the 1st test)
Two cortisol samples were a little below the reference limits
Total daily cortisol – 21.8 nmol/l   (Range 21–41)

5th and final Test   (20 months after the 1st test)
One remaining low cortisol level in the late afternoon
Total daily cortisol – 26.7 nmol/l   (Range 21–41)

Adrenal fatigue treatment – summary

Although Mrs X had obtained relief from her symptoms, she understood the wisdom of annual repeat adrenal tests. Unfortunately adrenal fatigue or insufficiency can develop very gradually, before a patient's warning symptoms begin to surface. The timescale and the results of the five tests provide tangible evidence for the therapeutic value of the adrenal glandular supplements that I prescribed. The results also demonstrate the time-scale of the condition and Mrs X's slow response to treatment that is so often part of CFS; it was only after almost two years of treatment that Mrs X felt her 'old self'.

The cost of treatment

At this stage you may well be thinking, 'What did all that cost?' Naturopathy is not a hands-on treatment; I do not need to see patients weekly, or even monthly. I usually recommend follow-up appointments for patients to see me initially after one month to discuss recent test results, and then perhaps every three to four month thereafter. In Mrs X's case, we only had a 'face-to-face' to discuss specific test results and to review treatment requirements. Over a two-year period, I saw her only seven times.

My standard recommendation to patients when I first see them is, 'Please make contact if questions or problems arise.' In recent years this has usually been by email or, occasionally, letters or telephone messages via my receptionists. CFS rarely includes acute symptoms, and the majority of patients who seek help have had their symptoms for several years. However, Mrs X's case demonstrated the value of patience (mine and hers) when treating CFS and allied conditions.

Barbara's story

At her first consultation, Barbara had symptoms of fibromyalgia, with chronic fatigue, joint pain and stiffness, which she had had for over three years. She was a 60-year-old self-employed shop owner with a long history of stress. Her stress load included a major road traffic accident, which had caused multiple fractures, 20 years previously, and chronic endometriosis which had been treated with a hysterectomy. She had also suffered before the hysterectomy from long-term heavy and painful periods. Recent hot flushes and raised blood pressure, sinus and chest congestion all added to her current symptoms.

Test results showed Barbara to have very mild hypothyroidism; however, I thought this could be a symptom of adrenal fatigue, the latter being confirmed in her first adrenal stress profile test. Her medical treatment to date had consisted of a low dose beta-blocker drug for high blood pressure and a trial on the HRT drug Premarin for the hot flushes. The Premarin proved to be ineffective and was discontinued. Unfortunately, the side-effects of the beta-blocker included fatigue, poor circulation to the limbs, breathlessness, headaches and insomnia.

Barbara's adrenal test confirmed adrenal exhaustion and chronic inefficiency. Her 'total daily cortisol' was a very low 7.2 nmol/l, the recommended normal range being 21–41 nmol/l. I recommended nutritional adrenal support and dietary advice and within eight months her total daily cortisol had increased to 12.9 with matching improvement in her symptoms.

Barbara was able to stop taking the beta-blocker and her improved stress handling and adrenal efficiency ensured that her blood pressure remained at a normal level. Her fatigue and joint symptoms improved over a two-year period and she was virtually symptom-free at her last visit. A final adrenal stress profile test showed a total daily cortisol of 25.4 nmol/l, which was her first 'normal' level in almost four years.

Two common and understandable questions asked by recovered patients are, 'What happens if my symptoms return?' and 'How will I know if my health is failing again?' This highlights the value of an annual maintenance check with a repeat adrenal test, and thyroid blood test if required. Once symptoms have improved and adrenal test results have confirmed that stress-handling has returned to normal, it is not difficult for a patient to be aware if his/her adrenal capacity is declining and symptoms are returning.

Adrenal fatigue – medical treatment

Medicine recognises two types of adrenal insufficiency: Addison's disease is known as 'primary'; the more common type is known as 'secondary' and is caused by problems with the pituitary gland or trauma to the head.

These types of adrenal insufficiency are usually treated with hydrocortisone. However, Plenadren is the first alternative medical treatment developed in more than 50 years. It provides a more gentle control of cortisol levels and fewer side-effects than does hydrocortisone.

Fibromyalgia

I have observed that patients with fibromyalgia symptoms often have a problem with cellular energy, coupled with low thyroid and adrenal status. When this is the case, I often find that guaifenesin is a valuable treatment.

Guaifenesin – a brief history

As early as 1553, the boiled tree bark named guaiacum was prescribed for rheumatism and gout. Although female gout is uncommon, many female sufferers of fibromyalgia have gout in the family. In the 1920s it was recommended for 'growing pains' in children and for fibrositis (fibromyalgia) symptoms. In the 1940s it was purified into 'guaiacolate' and prescribed in cough mixtures to reduce and thin mucous and phlegm.

Guaifenesin is now recommended in much larger doses to treat the symptoms of fibromyalgia by purging excess phosphate from the body. Oxalate and excess cellular calcium are also reduced. Excessive cellular phosphate interrupts energy (ATP) production, leading to pain and fatigue. Although phosphate is normally quite harmless, any excess in the wrong place can cause symptoms. Its removal can lead to a build-up of cellular debris via the kidneys, causing a *temporary* exacerbation of symptoms. This worsening has been termed 'reversal symptoms', which, although distressing to the patient, confirm that the guaifenesin therapy is working.

After the initial flare-up of symptoms, which should occur within two weeks, there can be subsequent repeated reversal symptoms, but they are rarely as severe as the initial response. This apparent worsening of symptoms is not a 'de-tox', as guaifenesin is non-toxic. Perhaps the term 'healing crisis' is more appropriate. If no reaction occurs, the usual procedure is to double the dosage.

Guaifenesin has no known side-effects, other than the reversal symptoms, and it can be taken with prescription drugs and supplements, apart from the salicylates, which I will now explain.

Salicylates – a brief history

Salts of salicylic acid (Salix willow) are medically prescribed as a pain killer.

Prescribed as an analgesic (pain killer) as early as 1800 BC, Hippocrates advised the bark of willow trees for aches and pains in 500 BC. During the 15th and 16th centuries, willow-bark medicine became so popular to relieve pain and fevers that it was outlawed to save the wicker industry. In 1823 the active chemical, salicin, was extracted from willow bark and many other plants and given the Latin name of *Salix*. A synthetic alternative was produced in 1899 and given the name of 'aspirin'.

Salicylates versus guaifenesin

It is essential to avoid all sources of salicylates if guaifenesin is to work for fibromyalgia symptoms. This is for the following reason. The development of drugs (pharmacology) is based on substances that can be successfully absorbed by our receptor cells, resulting in an action being either blocked or triggered. Unfortunately, guaifenesin and the salicylates compete for the same receptors in the kidney tubules, but the salicylates are a better fit. Guaifenesin will successfully treat mucous congestion in the lungs because the lung receptors are not compromised by circulating salicylates. However, its benefit in fibromyalgia is virtually non-existent if the patient takes aspirin-based medicines.

For many years, gout remedies have carried an 'avoid aspirin' warning on their labels, showing the conflict between the salicylates and guaifenesin was well known. However, it is only in recent years that it has become apparent that even small amounts of salicylates, absorbed through the skin, can cancel out the symptom relief from guaifenesin. Research has shown that tiny amounts of salicylates applied to the skin can be measured in almost the same concentration on the other side of the body, within 30 minutes. This means it is necessary to identify and avoid *all* sources of salicylates in cosmetics, medicines, dental products and, of course, food. Be aware that the blocking effect of the salicylates is cumulative – a little and often makes guaifenesin useless.

How to avoid salicylates

You need to avoid these ingredients:

- Salicylate and salicylic acid (including medicines and cosmetics – many products for acne, dandruff etc contain salicylic acid so read the ingredients)
- Acetyl-salicylic acid (sometimes abbreviated to ASA) – this is aspirin and is found in many combined analgesics
- Oil extracts or gels with a plant name (but *not* including soya, wheat, oats, rice and corn)
- Chemicals with names that include 'sal'
- Chemicals with names that include 'camph' and 'menth' – camphor and menthol are also classed as salicylates
- Bioflavonoids, quercetin, rutin and hesperidin
- Products with 'flavours', such as toothpaste, cough drops etc
- Mint of any kind (peppermint, spearmint etc)
- Pycnogenol, bisadol or balsam – (they are all from barks).

Natural sources of salicylates

All plants contain some salicylates, so avoid all herbal medications. Look out for plant names with the addition of oil, gel and extract. The concentrated plant pigments hesperiden, rutin and bioflavonoids will also block guaifenesin. Natural salicylates are found only in plants, never in mineral or animal products.

Smokers need to be aware that tobacco plants contain menthyl salicylate. Be on the safe side and avoid smoking.

Dietary sources of salicylates

Only the mint family must be avoided, plus tea. *Small* amounts of herbs are acceptable to flavour a recipe. Food when eaten in normal amounts will not block guaifenesin as the salicylates in food are partially destroyed by digestion.

Rita's story

Rita was 50 years old and had been suffering from CFS for a little over four years when she first came to see me. The symptoms developed shortly after a very stressful divorce, and included general fatigue that was worse on rising, poor memory and concentration, muscle/joint pain, chiefly in the back and neck, headaches and a degree of irritability. Rita also suffered bloating after meals and chronic constipation. She was self-employed, owning and running several shops. The only medical treatment she had been offered was anti-depressant drugs, which Rita refused to take. Her GP had decided that the cause of her symptoms was menopausal stress.

Although I thought it very likely from her fatigue and joint/muscle pain that Rita was suffering from the symptoms of fibromyalgia, I decided that routine testing for the causes of CFS was an appropriate first step in her diagnosis.

The results showed borderline hypothyroidism, a low 'total daily cortisol' and borderline low ferritin. A gut fermentation profile to identify candidiasis (see chapter 5, page 128) and an intestinal permeability profile to check for a possible 'leaky gut' (see page 129) were both normal. However, I also requested a CFS profile, which includes ATP activity. This showed low ATP and rapid depletion of ATP on increased energy demand. Rita's Acumen test results are shown in Figure 6.6 (see page 202).

Rita's treatment regime

I advised the following programme for Rita's reduced ATP activity: co-enzyme Q-10, L-carnitine, magnesium glycinate, NADH (B-3), ribose (a sugar that can convert quickly into ATP), and Hemagenics (iron bisglycinate). I also recommended thyroid and adrenal glandular, a plant-based digestive enzyme supplement, and omega-3 supplements. After three months, a follow-up Acumen test showed progress, but unfortunately Rita's symptoms were only slightly improved, so I considered it was worth trying guaifenesin.

Rita's response to guaifenesin

After a two-week trial on guaifenesin Rita experienced a symptom flare-up which confirmed that the treatment to reduce phosphates was worthwhile. Within four weeks, she was experiencing complete days without symptoms, and after three months she was improved by around 50% for all her symptoms.

Three months later Rita continued to take a maintenance dosage of guaifenesin but could stop taking her other supplements. I consider that further tests are necessary after six months for patients like Rita, assuming their symptom improvement continues.

Biolab Medical Unit

Gut Fermentation Profile

NOTE: A glucose load was given one hour before sampling.

	Result (µmol/1)	Reference Range:
Alcohols: In most cases, It is only the ethanol result that is affected by the glucose load.		
Ethanol	85	less than 22
	0.4 mg/dl	less than 0.1
Methanol	N.D.	less than 2.5
2-propanol	1.1	less than 1.0
1-propanol	2.5	less than 0.5
2-methyl-2-propanol	N.D.	less than 0.3
2-methyl-1-propanol	0.6	less than 0.3
2-butanol	1.5	less than 2.3
1-butanol	1.6	less than 1.2
2-methyl-2-butanol	N.D.	less than 0.5
2-methyl-1-butanol	0.6	less than 0.3
2-ethyl-1-butanol	6.2	less than 1.0
2,3 -butylene glycol	4.2	less than 2.5
Short chain fatty acids and related substances:		
Acetate	70	52–85
Propionate	34	10–56
Butyrate	12	7–33
Succinate	4	1–31
Valerate	11	2–19

N.D. = Not Detected.

Comment: All results assume 24 hours without alcohol ingestion and three to twelve hours fasting.

Figure 6.5: Rita's Acumen test results

Oxalates and fibromyalgia

Oxalates are non-toxic, naturally occurring substances, found in animals, plants and humans. Described as organic acid molecules, they are manufactured by animals and plants, or they result from the conversion of other substances, an example being vitamin C, which our cells can convert into oxalates. So, in summary, oxalates are either made by the body or are contained in certain foods.

Chapter 6

It is thought that oxalates, as oxalic crystals, are responsible for the pain and other symptoms of fibromyalgia. Chronic fatigue is a typical symptom of a high build-up of oxalate in the body, while chronic pain, hypothyroidism, asthma, cystic fibrosis, autism, muscle and joint stiffness, depression, and poor memory and concentration, can all be influenced by high oxalate levels. Specific symptoms of too much oxalate can include irritability, restless legs, muscular weakness and stiffness, involuntary twitching, insomnia, cystitis and irritable bowel syndrome.

The following are suspected of causing oxalate build-up:

1. Antibiotics, which tend to destroy the 'friendly' gut bacteria
2. Gut permeability disorders, such as 'leaky gut'
3. Problems with inefficient fat digestion
4. Very low-fat diets
5. High-carbohydrate diets: a low-carbohydrate diet can be a successful treatment for oxalate-related symptoms, including fibromyalgia. Meat, with fat included, is of special value.

Sufferers of oxalate build-up are chiefly middle-aged women. One explanation for this may be that dietary oxalate is not normally absorbed by the body, but the lower oestrogen linked to menopause may allow more oxalate to pass into the body. It can form crystals and contribute to the fibromyalgia-type symptoms of muscle, bladder and brain as previously defined. Significantly, the treatment of fibromyalgia with guaifenesin can cause a 30% increase in oxalate excretion, in addition to the phosphate and calcium removal.

Oxalate has been described as a 'waste product' excreted in the urine. Unfortunately, it can cause irritation and burning in the tissues that the urine passes through. This can cause cystitis and vulvar pain (vulvodynia). Such symptoms are frequently mis-diagnosed as candidiasis, urinary infections or food allergies.

A more serious condition linked to too much oxalate in the diet is kidney stones. Approximately 80% of stones are composed of calcium oxalate. There is no effective test for oxalate excess, except for urine oxalate measurement, used in the diagnosis of possible kidney stones.

Diets low in oxalate and calcium are prescribed to reduce the risk of stones forming (see the list of foods to avoid below), but the relationship between dietary oxalate and kidney stone formation is controversial. Many researchers doubt the value of complete avoidance. However, there is evidence that oxalate-rich foods can cause and aggravate fibromyalgia-type symptoms. For this reason, a low-oxalate diet may be worthwhile for patients following the guaifenesin treatment programme to treat fibromyalgia.

Foods containing oxalates

Oxalate is present at the highest levels in plants; the lists below should be a useful guide. Some sufferers are very sensitive to certain oxalate-rich foods, suffering rapid symptom 'flare-ups' similar to responses to allergens in foods.

Coffee, tea, cocoa, chocolate, beer, soy milk
Nuts, all types
Wheat germ (cereals and brown bread)
Berries (black berries and berries of all types)
Fruit (rhubarb, tangerines, plums, black grapes)
Vegetables (beans, sesame seeds, sunflower seeds, spinach, leeks, celery, swede and soya beans)
Sardines (especially tinned)

You should also reduce the amount of salt, sugar and vitamin C you use, and drink plenty of water.

NB – When strict avoidance of oxalate is recommended, food sources should be limited to around 50 milligrams per day. An example of a food source containing 50 milligrams of oxalate would be ¼ cup of raw spinach. Assuming no other food source on the same day, this would represent the upper limit for oxalate in the diet.

Low-oxalate safe foods

Food selection with low-oxalate 'diets' is often based on individual responses to certain specific foods. Levels are low in the following list:

Dairy products – Cheese, milk, yoghurt and white chocolate
Proteins – turkey, chicken, lamb, pork and beef; eggs; fish (except sardines)
Vegetables – cauliflower, mushrooms, onions (but avoid spring onions), peas, cucumber, courgettes, white cabbage

Fruit – bananas, cherries, pears, coconut, papaya, white grapes, mangoes, apples, melon, honey

Condiment and oils – white pepper, vegetable oil (but avoid sunflower and sesame oils)

Drinks – wine, spirits, milk.

Oxalates and cooking – Cooking all types of foods has very little effect (good or bad) on the oxalate content, although boiling or steaming vegetables has been found to reduce their oxalate content by up to 10%. The loss of minerals and vitamins resulting from such overcooking (particularly of green vegetables) will tend to counteract any benefit obtained from the very slight oxalate loss.

NB: Those who have a tendency to form calcium oxalate in their urine improve by up to 15% with a strict oxalate restriction diet. The words 'limited' or 'reduced' are frequently used to define oxalate-rich foods, in such diets, rather than 'total avoidance'.

Low-oxalate diets – summary
A high vegetable diet can cause an excess of oxalates in the body, particularly if there is an emphasis on soya-based food to provide protein. Nuts and seeds are also high in oxalates.

Trying a low-oxalate diet
In the absence of a definitive test to diagnose oxalate disorders, and the suspected role of oxalate build-up in fibromyalgia, trying out a low-oxalate diet can be a safe and effective route to a diagnosis and possible symptom relief. If you decide to follow a low-oxalate diet, you will need to turn a blind eye to the medical dogma that has surfaced in recent years concerning what constitutes a 'healthy diet'. These include the following *false* guidelines:

1. Eat plenty of fruit and vegetables – five portions daily is considered ideal
2. Bran and fibre are always good for us and wholemeal brown bread and cereal are therefore better than the white equivalent
3. If you eat chocolate, go for the dark variety; its higher cacao content can assist control of your blood pressure

4. Vitamin C is always a good remedy for colds and other infections
5. Vegetarianism is a healthy option; most of us eat too much animal protein. Soya products are a healthy plant protein in preference to meat
6. The ideal healthy diet should be high in complex carbohydrates
7. Fruit of all types should be an important component in our daily diet.

None of these so-called guidelines for health apply to a low-oxalate diet. But do not worry – if you have a potential oxalate problem, avoiding high-oxalate foods should be the priority. As with so many nutritional treatments and specialised diets, there is no such thing as a standard response. I usually advise patients to follow the diet and allow three months to assess any worthwhile improvement in symptoms.

It has been observed that the oxalate content can vary between plants of the same species. Differences in climate, soil type, and other factors play a part. As I described above, a low-oxalate diet is usually based on consuming less than 50 milligrams of total oxalate daily. The low-oxalate foods I have listed above are usually seen as guidelines for patients with suspected or an actual history of kidney stones.

If there is no noticeable symptom-relief after 10 to 12 weeks of this exclusion diet, then oxalate build-up is unlikely to be a factor contributing to your symptoms.

You may wish to seek further information online. This can be reassuring and helpful. Unfortunately, the food lists and diets do not always follow standardised patterns. You may have to do some research (see www.lowoxalate.info (UK) and www.litholink.com (USA)).

Candidiasis

I have discussed the part candidiasis may play in CFS in chapter 3 (see page 59), and looked at diagnosis in chapter 5 (see page 128). In this chapter I am reviewing treatment. To illustrate treatment of candidiasis in the context of chronic fatigue, I have included 'Rose's story' (see below). Although this includes a treatment programme, this section calls for more detail regarding the general treatment of candidiasis.

Inevitably, when candidiasis is diagnosed, the first priority is to review and where necessary amend a patient's diet. I very rarely meet patients whose sole problem is candidiasis. Many show symptoms of a 'leaky gut', enzyme deficiencies and irritable bowel-type symptoms. Whatever else is going wrong with a person's health, if systemic candidiasis has been diagnosed, a logical first step is to follow a low-sugar, low-alcohol and yeast-free diet, either for three to four months, or until a follow-up gut fermentation test (the test for candida – see page 128) can confirm a normal, candida-free response.

Diet for candida control
Foods to avoid
This is a diet low in sugar, alcohol and yeast, so the following must be avoided:

Sugar in all forms and all bread and flour products (such as cakes and biscuits) *except* yeast-free unleavened bread

Alcohol in all forms

Citrus juices unless freshly squeezed

Malt drinks

Nuts, unless freshly cracked and in season (otherwise yeasts can be a problem)

Cereals containing added vitamins and malt

All dried fruits

Fungi, mushrooms and moulds (such as in blue cheeses)

Foods containing monosodium glutamate

Cheese, *except* for a little mild white English cheese

Buttermilk and yoghurt with added vitamins

Anything fried in breadcrumbs, such as fish fingers

Meat extracts (OXO, Marmite etc)

Hamburgers, sausages, smoked fish and meat

Condiments and pickles, salad dressings, sauerkraut, olives, chillies etc

Vitamin B complex, except those prescribed by someone who knows you are trying to control candida.

All fruits and vegetables should be as fresh as possible, and in season for where you are (that is, nothing imported, like strawberries in December if you are in the northern hemisphere). They should also be well washed before use.

You should drink *still* mineral water only.

Your environment is important too. If possible avoid damp atmospheres and old buildings that may support moulds and rot, such as cellars, old clothes and books. Use only freshly laundered towels; damp towels encourage mould growth.

Supplements to help candida control

Although patients' requirements can vary, I tend to prescribe a standard supplement list to treat candidiasis and support the diet. This includes a high potency formula to treat candidia and support gut microbe balance. This is Nutrispore™ by Nutri Advanced, which consists of the following:

Caprylic acid	Black walnut hulls powder
Garlic	Beet (root)
Cinnamon (bark)	Aloe vera (leaf)
Thyme (leaf)	Grapefruit (seed) extract
Basil (leaf)	Clove (flower bud)
Undecylenic acid	Oregano (leaf)
Turmeric extract	Zinc (picolinate).

Probiotics help to support beneficial gut bacteria. The Nutri Probiotic Plus formula contains an exclusive blend of probiotics and provides 750 million viable organisms per capsule. Lactobacillus and Bifidobacterium have been complemented by five additional bacterial strains, including *Lactobacillus rhamnosus* and *Lactobacillus plantarum*, which provide an excellent blend for an optimal bacterial micro-environment in the large intestine. The precise ingredients are:

Beta-galactosidase
Bacterial powder providing: *B. bifidum, L. acidophilus, L. rhamnosus, B. longum, B. infantis, B. adolescentis, L. plantarum*
Amylase
Cellulase.

Anti-candidiasis herbals

The following herbs possess known antifungal properties. They are usually sold as teas, but they can also be used as douches or tampon soakings for vaginitis.

Aloe vera (useful as a douche)	Sorbis (mountain ash cream, sold as
Chamomile	Cervagyn)
Berberine	Tea tree oil.

In addition, acidophilus culture can be effective when inserted vaginally, particularly when diluted with a little aloe vera juice. Garlic is also a valuable anti-candida herb, taken orally.

Medical treatment for candidiasis

It is ironic that the usual medical prescription for candida treatment is the anti-fungal drug nystatin, which is itself yeast based. When taken it can show a characteristic 'rebound effect' – a noticeable worsening of yeast colonies in the gut, often more than before treatment commenced. Caprylic acid does not show this rebound effect. Although nystatin is largely non-toxic, its side-effects are thought to result from the massive destruction of the candida. This stresses the immune system and the body's response to the breakdown products.

Candidiasis treatment – summary

The common yeast *Candida albicans* is in all of us. Normally it is harmless. Unfortunately, the modern use of antibiotics can kill off the beneficial bacteria which help keep candidia in check. As with yeast-free B-complex formulae, it was quite normal practice when antibiotics were first prescribed in the 1940s and 1950s to include an anti-fungal drug in the prescription. This is no longer recommended.

There are other causes of candidia overgrowth; these can include:

Anti-ulcer drugs
Oral contraceptives (birth control)
Steroids
Faulty or deficient digestive acid and enzymes
Excessive alcohol
Excessive sugar.

There is little doubt, in spite of the above list, that the huge increase in yeast infections over the previous half-century can be largely put down to over-enthusiastic antibiotic use.

Rose's story

When she first came to see me, Rose was a 46-year-old housewife, suffering from multiple food allergies, fatigue and almost constant cystitis and indigestion. It was quite clear to me that her very limited diet, a result of her food intolerances, was just one of her many problems. For more than 20 years she had suffered with stomach fullness, flatulence and morning diarrhoea. In addition, after several courses of broad spectrum antibiotics for her repeated throat infections, she admitted that she 'caught every infection doing the rounds'. Other symptoms included pre-menstrual syndrome, frequent headaches, sore throats and poor memory and concentration. She was a depressed, anxious person who was concerned that her current health was worsening.

She was relying more and more on various drugs for symptom-relief. She had been given a diagnosis of a poor immune system, irritable bowel syndrome and depression by her GP.

It is very tempting for practitioners to offer symptom-relief treatments to their CFS patients. However, I consider that a check-list of the most likely possible causes must be compiled as an essential first step in understanding their complaint. A clear separation of causes and symptoms can be a crucial aid to diagnosis. With many of the CFS patients who consult me, it is apparent that for many years only their symptoms have been treated. With the passage of time, this approach can so often lead to a worsening of the underlying causes and thereby of the symptoms.

Rose's past treatment had included antibiotics, anti-depressants, prednisolone (cortisone), antacids and anti-fungal creams. Her GP had tested her for iron-deficient anaemia, vitamin B-12 deficiency and a thyroid hormone profile. In addition to these standard medical tests, I requested tests to measure a possible 'leaky gut' – the intestinal permeability (or PEG) test (see page 129). This involves taking urine samples over a six-hour period and can indicate the possibility of an increase in gut permeability. I also requested a gut fermentation test, which specifically identifies the presence and severity of candidiasis. It achieves this by measuring the amount of ethanol (alcohol) in a patient's blood 60 minutes after ingesting a measured amount of glucose. As brewers are well aware, glucose plus yeast equals alcohol. The amount of alcohol in a patient's blood following ingestion of glucose can therefore clearly show the presence of yeast – that is, *Candida albicans*. Rose tested positive to this test, confirming the presence of a yeast colony in her intestines. This was a likely cause of her leaky gut.

As I described in chapter 5 (Diagnosis) the tests for candidiasis and leaky gut are not available on the NHS. They are tests provided by a specialised private laboratory in central London named Biolab.

I have included an analysis detailing the flaws in Rose's original medical diagnosis. This serves to demonstrate why she suffered from CFS symptoms for 30 long years.

1. Her blood tests for vitamin B-12, iron reserves (ferritin) and thyroid status were all within the standard (very low) normal ranges but only just; they were all borderline low and as a result no treatment was offered.

2. Candidiasis is not recognised in mainstream medicine as a systemic condition, but rather as a local problem of the throat or vagina. The treatment offered is usually a prescription for anti-fungal creams. GPs have been known to refer their suspected candida patients to gynaecologists. Antibiotics were prescribed for Rose's cystitis, which is a sure-fire way to worsen candidiasis.

3. Although allergy testing had confirmed a genuine intolerance to cows' milk and avoidance was advised, no other nutritional advice was recommended. Unfortunately, the simple avoidance of cows' milk did not improve any of Rose's symptoms.

4. The concept of a leaky gut is not an accepted syndrome in medicine. Therefore it is not fully understood or treated.

5. The importance of the beneficial bacteria (probiotics) is also not addressed in medical diagnosis or treatment. When candida is caused by excessive antibiotic use, the beneficial gut bacteria can be seriously reduced, thus allowing the 'bad guys' to proliferate in the gut, contributing to a leaky gut.

6. The majority of Rose's symptoms were diagnosed as 'pre-menopausal' by her GP. These symptoms included pre-menstrual syndrome with moodiness, sugar-craving and weight increase as a result of fluid retention, reduced libido, fatigue, depression, poor immunity, morning headaches and joint and muscle pain and stiffness.

7. The treatment of antacids served to aggravate an existing low stomach acid (hypochlorhydria).

Many of Rose's symptoms were typical of candidiasis but were discounted by her GP in favour of a pre-menstrual explanation; female hormones were blamed for many of Rose's symptoms.

In addition to investigating leaky gut and candidiasis, I also requested an adrenal function saliva test that showed profoundly low cortisol levels. Details of this test and a comparison with the standard medical tests for adrenal status are discussed earlier in the book (see page 121).

Rose's story shows how often chronic fatigue can be the result of several causes. Her central problem may well have been systemic candidiasis, which gave rise to many of her symptoms, psychological and physical. However, her depressed metabolism, poor digestion and absorption, the resulting stress and poorly balanced diet all contributed to her fatigue.

The vicious circle of stress, lethargy, mood changes and many other symptoms, resulting in additional stress, is a symptom pattern frequently observed in my CFS patients. In spite of her long and complex history of poor health, Rose's diagnosis after seeing various medical specialists and undergoing many tests, can be summarised as follows: a neurotically depressed, pre-menopausal patient, with poor immunity, IBS (irritable bowel syndrome) and food allergies.

Rose's treatment programme

My first priority when preparing a treatment strategy for CFS patients is to prescribe the appropriate treatment for any obvious, easily identified deficiencies. For Rose this meant iron supplements coupled with a diet that included iron-rich foods, a course of vitamin B-12 intra-muscular injections to 'top-up' her low blood B-12, and thyroid glandular supplements to boost her thyroid output. Significantly, these three areas of borderline low function are all known to cause fatigue as a common symptom. A course of hydrochloric acid tablets to assist Rose's digestive symptoms was also prescribed.

As far as Rose's candidiasis was concerned, the first step was to advise a sugar-free, refined-carbohydrate-free and yeast-free diet and to avoid alcohol. I recommended a high dosage caprylic acid supplement, this being a short-chain fatty acid and a derivative of coconut oil. It is an effective and safe supplement to reduce yeast overgrowth in the gut. With candidiasis, our body's B vitamins can be reduced. When discussing prescribing customs with older GPs it always interests me to learn that it was customary in the late 1940s and the 1950s to prescribe antibiotics coupled with a vitamin B complex. The link between antibiotics and candidiasis potentially reducing several B vitamins in the gut was recognised. Unfortunately, this is no longer considered significant, so B-complex tablets are no longer prescribed or recommended.

Deficiencies in vitamins A and C, zinc and magnesium can also compromise gut health. I therefore advised Rose to take a comprehensive multi-vitamin formula and a high dosage vitamin B complex (rice-based *not* yeast-based).

As beneficial gut bacteria are reduced in candidiasis, I also prescribed a course of probiotics, these being friendly bacteria which normally support bacterial balance in the large intestine. These can also be found in natural yoghurts, but high dosage probiotics in capsule form are often essential.

A second series of tests after three months of treatment showed all-round improvement. This matched Rose's declared symptom relief. Her increased mental and physical energy had encouraged her to face the future more optimistically.

There are close links between systemic candidiasis, food and environmental intolerances and our histamine status. CFS has rightly been defined as a symptom complex. Rose's symptoms and her improvement subsequent to treatment served to confirm my view that CFS is rarely simple exhaustion.

Food intolerance

As I have outlined earlier (see pages 63 and 176), food allergies and intolerances can be a major influence in causing CFS. While I have made it clear throughout the book that I do not recognise single causes for the complexity of CFS, any condition that compromises food digestion and absorption must be suspect as a contributory cause. Certainly, adverse reactions (allergies) to common foods are often involved.

Cathy's story

When she first came to see me, Cathy was a 24-year-old single mother with a long history of fatigue, coupled with almost constant indigestion and repeated throat infections. Her digestive symptoms consisted of stomach fullness and cramping, and diarrhoea with mild nausea. Cathy was also depressed and suffered morning headaches and heartburn or reflux. Past treatments had consisted of antacids, and anti-depressants. She had been diagnosed with IBS (irritable bowel syndrome) and stress symptoms.

Her diet was not ideal, being based on a 'little and often' regime. Unfortunately, her snacks were usually carbohydrate-based convenience foods, with very limited nutritional value. With the almost constant diarrhoea and stomach cramping that occurred two to three hours after eating, she had decided to eat frequently, hoping to avoid symptoms. Unfortunately, this plan did not work, making her even more depressed.

Her symptoms of fatigue (worse on rising), depression and poor immunity were typical symptoms of poor digestion. If we do not efficiently convert our food into energy, then fatigue is inevitable. I considered there was a real possibility of a food intolerance, which was confirmed when she mentioned that eating dairy foods always made her diarrhoea worse. Although it was tempting simply to categorise Cathy as a neurotic, inadequate young women suffering from many symptoms caused by stress, I suspected that her depression and fatigue were secondary to her faulty digestion and poor diet.

Cathy's diagnosis

I decided to request an adrenal stress profile. This confirmed adrenal fatigue. Her reduced adrenal function contributed to her morning symptoms and low blood sugar with low cortisol levels.

Cathy had been tested for *Helicobacter pylori*, the bacterium thought to be responsible for high stomach acid and stomach ulcers; this had shown negative results. In spite of this, Cathy had been advised to take antacid tablets for several years.

With her sensitivity to dairy products, I considered that Cathy was lactose (milk sugar) intolerant. This occurs when the digestive enzyme lactase is deficient and results in an inability to digest the lactose sugar that is present in all dairy products. Symptoms can include diarrhoea and abdominal cramping and discomfort. With chronic diarrhoea, nutrients are inadequately absorbed adding to the fatigue.

Cathy's treatment

I prescribed a supplement to increase Cathy's stomach acidity and thereby reduce her stomach fullness after meals. In addition, I placed Cathy on a dairy exclusion diet, coupled with strict avoidance of sugar and all refined carbohydrates (cakes, biscuits, etc). The supplements I advised included a high dosage vitamin/mineral compound, and adrenal glandulars.

Within two weeks Cathy's diarrhoea and stomach cramps had eased and she began to feel less fatigued, particularly on rising. After further improvement in her symptoms and total avoidance of dairy products for six weeks, I allowed her to re-introduce dairy foods. Moreover, I supplied lactase tablets to be taken immediately before she had food or drink containing milk. This provided her missing digestive enzyme and she no longer reacted to milk in her diet.

Cathy's story highlights the importance of diet and digestive efficiency in people with CFS. There may not be evidence of a defined disorder or disease, but poor digestion is a frequently missed but contributing cause of chronic fatigue.

Low blood sugar (hypoglycaemia)

Mainstream medicine has assumed for many years that low blood sugar is seen only as a symptom of a diabetic 'hypo', this being the result of a misjudged insulin dosage by an insulin-dependent diabetic causing blood sugar to fall below the normal minimum of 4 mmol/l. However, I and colleagues have seen many patients with episodes of low blood sugar who were *not* diabetic. In some cases, the level fell as low as 2 mmol/l. The chief symptom of low blood sugar is fatigue, particularly on rising or with missed meals. The problem is often associated with a history of stress and being overweight. The following case history will detail a typical diagnostic and treatment protocol for low blood sugar.

Sam's story

When Sam first consulted me he was a self-employed painter and decorator aged 31 years. The symptoms he described included: fatigue (worse on rising), aching muscles, poor memory and concentration, overweight by around 3 stone (42 pounds or 19 kilos), indigestion with fullness and stomach wind after meals, persistent sugar cravings, extreme hunger if missing meals, and anxiety attacks with depression. Many of these symptoms had been with him for more than 10 years. He admitted to disliking company and tended to be anti-social. He also had headaches (worse in the morning) almost daily, together with severe loss of confidence. He tended to be a self-confessed 'control freak' and perfectionist.

Sam's diet was not good; he ate chocolate bars three to four times each day and drank between four to five litres of sweet squash daily. His symptoms and diet pointed to a possible blood sugar problem. However, his symptoms had persisted through most of his adult life, from the age of 12 years, so I decided to 'dig deep' and requested thyroid function and adrenal function tests.

The adrenal stress profile (saliva test) showed a very low level of cortisol on getting up in the morning, and at the end of the day. His DHEA level was also too low. This suggested long-standing stressors and depleted levels of vital adrenal hormones.

The thyroid blood test profile showed a low free T4 (thyroxine) level, well below a normal range for his age. I recommended that Sam purchase a glucometer (easily available from a high street chemist) and to check his blood sugar on rising and when he experienced his daily sugar cravings. This he did and the readings showed a pronounced tendency to low blood sugar, with several results below 4 mmol/l.

Although Sam's diet was not seriously poor, it was high in sugar and as he had his last meal at 19.00 hours, it was followed by a 12-hour period without food each night. With his adrenal fatigue and subsequent poor blood sugar control, it meant that he was waking each day with hypoglycaemia, as was confirmed by the glucometer checks.

I prescribed a low-sugar diet, as described below, coupled with thyroid and adrenal glandular supplements, including DHEA.

Diet for low blood sugar

On rising

A small glass of fresh fruit juice (a good pick-me-up) or beverage or small sugar-free natural yoghurt.

Breakfast

The ideal breakfast is a wholegrain cereal or one slice of wholemeal bread and sugar-free jam or marmalade. Fresh fruit. Sugar-free muesli can be purchased or homemade. For additional protein use sugar-free soya milk on the cereal. (Soya milk is more palatable when diluted 25% with water or fruit juice.)

If appetite allows select from the following: egg (scrambled, poached, boiled or omelette), low-sugar baked beans, sugar-free ham or grilled lean bacon, cheese on toast, sardines on toast, grilled or steamed fish with one slice of wholemeal bread (may be toasted) or brown rice. Roll and butter.

Two hours after breakfast

As on rising.

Lunch

- Meat, fish, cheese or eggs, salad (large serving of lettuce, tomato etc, with French dressing or mayonnaise), vegetables if desired. Only one slice of wholemeal bread, toast or crisp bread with butter
- Dessert – cheese, yoghurt or fruit
- Beverage.

Two hours after lunch (and every two hours until the evening meal)

As on rising.

Dinner

- Soup if desired; vegetables or salad; liberal portion of meat, fish or poultry; only one slice of wholemeal bread, if desired
- Dessert – cheese, yoghurt or fruit
- Beverage.

Two hours after dinner (and every two hours until supper)
As on rising.

Supper (as late as possible)
- Crisp bread with butter and pâté, cheese, ham or cold meat
- Beverage or milk; natural yoghurt.

Notes
- Dinner and lunch may be reversed
- Soya and other plant proteins make excellent substitutes for milk
- Avoid wherever possible the use of sugar substitutes
- Fruit and vegetables – avoid excess dates, raisins and bananas
- Beverage – restrict to any natural coffee substitute or decaffeinated coffee; or to herb teas or weak China or Indian teas
- Alcohol – if it does not cause symptoms, limit to one glass of dry white wine with dinner
- Soft drinks – 'sugar-free' soft drinks should be used very cautiously
- Tobacco – to be avoided, as should smoky atmospheres; each cigarette smoked raises the smoker's blood sugar by the equivalent of two and a half teaspoons of sugar
- Avoid – all products containing sugar (glucose, fructose, sucrose, dextrose, syrup, molasses, honey, etc). When eating cereal, bread, rice or pasta, obtain good-quality naturally produced wholemeal or wholegrain products.

I also advised Sam to take the GTF Complex™ (glucose tolerance factor) that I had designed for Nutri Advanced to assist blood sugar control. The GTF Complex™ comprises:

Magnesium	N-acetyl-cysteine	Zinc
Vitamin C	Vitamin B-3	Vitamin B-12
Potassium	Inositol	Pituitary glandular
Calcium	Vitamin B-6	Chromium
Vitamin E	Vitamin B-1	Parotid glandular
Pantothenic acid	Manganese	Folic acid
Choline	Vitamin B-2	Biotin
Adrenal concentrate	PABA (para-aminobenzoic acid)	

Within three months, Sam's morning lethargy was beginning to improve and he was consuming less sugar in his diet. Within six months, Sam was more or less as he hoped to be, being alert on rising and with a surplus of energy. His general memory and concentration had also improved, as had his social life. However, as his symptoms had been with him for many years, I considered that a maintenance treatment programme was appropriate, consisting of a low dosage supplement, a good diet and annual tests to ensure all was well.

Low blood sugar is often a symptom of a long-term health problem. Adrenal exhaustion, malabsorption, syndrome X and many other conditions can cause low blood sugar symptoms. However, as with Sam, it can also be the chief cause of symptoms.

Post-viral fatigue syndrome (PVFS)

'Post-viral fatigue syndrome' (PVFS) has become interchangeable with the term 'myalgic encephalomyelitis'. It has also been called 'Royal Free disease' following an outbreak of ME-type symptoms amongst staff and a few patients at the Royal Free Hospital, London, in July 1955.

'Post-viral fatigue syndrome' means simply a complex group of symptoms following a viral infection. This is where controversy and confusion take over. Simply because post-viral symptoms are recognised and typically follow a bout of 'flu, infective hepatitis or glandular fever, why are the symptoms that follow these conditions excluded from the PVFS group? This may be because there has been a tendency to assume that PVFS results from an undiscovered virus (recently disproved – see chapter 1, page 40). Or perhaps the answer lies in the duration of the symptoms: many practitioners and researchers believe that PVFS symptoms need to be present for at least six months before a diagnosis can be made.

Another major area of dispute regarding the causes and symptoms of PVFS is the widely held view that ME and PVFS, and even CFS, are expressions of hysteria and panic – the explanation given for the Royal Free epidemic. (Although a little under 300 members of staff were affected by the illness, strangely, in spite of the hospital being at full capacity, only 12 patients succumbed to the symptoms. Unfortunately many of the staff panicked at the rapid spread of the 'mysterious illness', which served to support the hypothesis of 'mass hysteria' that was later reported as a possible cause.)

A quotation from Celia Wookey's book *Myalgic Encephalomyelitis* published in 1986 demonstrates the alternative explanation for some of the symptoms: 'Symptoms like depression, insomnia and loss of concentration and memory which impair mental powers may be resented, but although they are psychological symptoms, they are caused by an organic virus infection of the brain and spinal cord. So are the mood-swings which are such a distressing symptom for many patients, particularly if combined with agitation or undue irritability.'

This serves to highlight the two different diagnostic explanations for the psychological symptoms common to PVFS and ME (depression, anxiety, irritability etc):

1. Psychological changes and symptoms *cause* the condition
2. Psychological symptoms result *from* the condition

Physical or psychological cause – summary
Having been consulted by many CFS patients who have experienced distressing mental and physical symptoms, I am never in doubt that the physical symptoms are first on the scene, followed by and causing the mental symptoms. These usually include depression, anxiety, and concentration and memory problems.

I see post-viral fatigue as an occasional contributory factor in explaining CFS. The initial enthusiasm for a viral explanation for CFS stemmed from outbreaks in the 1930s and 1940s. These were thought to be variants of poliomyelitis, in many cases being diagnosed as 'epidemic neuromyasthnia'. Significantly, only a few of the hundreds of cases reported at the time were described as psychogenic (that is, of the mind). As Valerie's story (see below) demonstrates, I believe that when young Europeans travel extensively in the Far East, they run the risk of developing a bacterial, or viral, reaction which subsequently leads to CFS.

Valerie's story

Valerie was a single woman of 24 years when she first came to see me. Working as a PA, her lifestyle was stressful and tiring. However, it was clear her chronic fatigue was out of proportion with her workload and life-style. She claimed to have been very fatigued for a little over three years. Her exhaustion and other symptoms had developed following a four-month holiday in Thailand. Her other symptoms included the following:

Dysmenorrhoea (period pain)
Menorrhagia (heavy periods)
Pre-menstrual syndrome (PMS) with dizziness and sugar-cravings
Severe heat rashes with exposure to sunlight
Very reduced libido (sex drive)
Poor immunity, constant colds, sinusitis and rhinitis
Stomach cramp and fullness after meals
Depressed, anxious and irritable, especially before periods and on rising.

Prior to her holiday in Thailand, Valerie had been quite fit and healthy. The only symptom that had concerned her was pre-menstrual headaches and general lethargy on rising. She had experienced quite a stressful childhood with bullying at school and divorced parents.

Although Valerie, upon her return from Thailand, had not immediately shown signs and symptoms of a specific complaint, it seemed clear to me that her immune system had suffered a set-back during her four-month holiday. Such a blow to the immune system is generally described as post-viral fatigue.

Our immune system works in close liaison with our system for handling stress. Fatigue or under-functioning of our adrenal system can compromise our blood sugar control, leading to low blood sugar (hypoglycaemia). The main symptoms resulting from this cascade of problems can include fatigue, infections, headaches, and anxiety with depression. Such symptoms can in themselves cause additional fatigue and anxiety, and a vicious circle is often established. When this occurs, possible causes and symptoms can become difficult to identify. This can result in the treatment prescribed being often based entirely upon symptom-relief, such as anti-depressants, antibiotics, short-term tonics and analgesics (pain killers).

Whatever happened to Valerie's metabolism during her stay in the Far East, it was clear that her immune system had been seriously compromised and after three years her symptoms still persisted. Unfortunately, Valerie had been taking a 'combined contraceptive' pill for four years. The chief side-effects of this particular pill include nausea, headaches, stomach cramps, depression and skin problems. I therefore advised her to discuss alternatives with her GP. The options were either to discontinue the pill for three to four months or, perhaps better, to request a progesterone-only contraceptive, these having fewer side-effects and being less inclined to trigger migraine attacks.

Valerie's treatment

I requested blood tests and an adrenal function stress profile. The results provided useful clues to Valerie's chronic fatigue. They showed borderline low levels of vitamin B-12 and ferritin (iron stores) and a low level for the thyroid hormone thyroxine (free T4). In addition, her adrenal hormones were also reduced, with low cortisol and DHEA levels.

Valerie had for over 10 years chosen to avoid red meat, eating only fish and chicken for her protein foods. Her previous heavy periods and red meat avoidance had depleted her iron stores (ferritin) and vitamin B-12 level. Both iron and vitamin B-12 are chiefly found in red meat. I therefore advised Valerie to eat red meat at least twice weekly and provided her with information on iron-rich foods. Although her anaemias were not severe, they contributed, with several other factors, to her stubborn CFS symptoms.

To complete the treatment, I advised Valerie to take the following supplements:

adrenal and thyroid glandular
vitamin B-12 with the intrinsic factor and supporting B vitamins
iron with synergistic DHEA
a two-phased (stomach and small bowel) digestive enzyme (such as
    Similase by Nutri Avanced)
a high-strength multi-mineral supplement.

I felt sure that her poor immunity and stress-handling were linked to her depressed thyroid/adrenal function, coupled with the anaemia. The side-effects of the contraceptive pill also may have contributed to her symptoms.

After a period of three months, Valerie began to make progress in all areas. However, her complete recovery took another six months of treatment. Her story shows how complex the causes of CFS can be and what the recovery time scale may be for CFS patients.

I am often asked by patients, 'How long will it take before I begin to feel better?' All I can say is that in my experience beneficial changes usually show after three to four months of treatment. However, full recovery is never guaranteed and long-term 'maintenance' treatment is often necessary. One of my colleagues has an approximate 'rule of thumb' for recovery time, that being a month for a year. This suggests that a chronic health problem that has lasted for six years may take six months before there is noticeable improvement in a patient's symptoms.

Valerie's story – summary

Valerie's case history serves to highlight the typical complexity of cause and effect in chronic fatigue, and the part played by post-viral fatigue, which often results from overseas travel. With many patients, there is a trigger that starts the symptoms. In Valerie's case this was her visit to Thailand. There was little doubt that her background health had not been good, and her avoidance of animal protein had contributed to her low vitamin B-12 and iron levels. Her heavy periods and the side-effects of her birth-control pill had contributed to the breakdown in her stamina and general health. The visit to Thailand constituted the last straw for her already poor health. So often a gap-year after college or university can cause real health problems in this way.

The symptoms of CFS can dramatically and suddenly worsen, when a person's metabolism is under stress and the energy reserve is low. An important clue to CFS in young patients is the loss of or reduction in their libido. Many regard this as a trivial symptom, but I believe it is a symptom that indicates very low stamina.

Haemochromatosis (referred to as 'H')

It has been suggested that medical terms are difficult to spell, and have been designed chiefly to keep patients confused and in ignorance. This description fits the term for 'iron overload' – that is, 'haemochromatosis' or 'H'. I have described this condition in chapter 4 (see page 85), and questioned the assumption that it is rare. I am currently seeing three patients with blood ferritin in excess of 400 µg/l (micrograms per litre), this being the level above which H may be diagnosed.

There are two chief types of iron overload disease: primary hereditary forms and various secondary forms.

Primary H

There are several different genetic mutations that can cause hereditary primary H. These can be identified in blood tests. More than 80% of primary H results from gene mutations. These cause increased and inappropriate iron absorption in the small intestine and, subsequently, increased iron storage in affected organs, including the liver, heart, pancreas and adrenal glands. Clinical problems resulting from this effect can include diabetes, cirrhosis of the liver, arthropathy (joint diseases), cardiomyopathy (heart disorders) and impotence.

Ferritin levels above 400 µg/l are seen as diagnostically significant. However, levels above 700 µg/l are frequently seen by practitioners.

Secondary H

Secondary H occurs over a lengthy period of time. The causes included excessive iron intake, taken as either oral supplements or by intra-muscular injection. Iron infusions and blood transfusions have in the past led to iron overload. To quote a respected medical textbook, *Clinical Aspects and Laboratory – Iron Metabolism, Anemias – concepts in the anemias of malignancies and renal and rheumatoid diseases* by M Wick, W Pinggera and P Lehman (2011): 'Iron overloading caused by transfusions should belong firmly to the past.'

Chronic alcoholism can also lead to secondary H, particularly in the presence of chronic liver disease. Although we tend to see lack of iron as being one of the main reasons for fatigue (that is, iron-deficient anaemia) it is quite clear that we can have 'too much of a good thing' and suffer symptoms resulting from iron overload. The key diagnostic test for high and low levels of iron should be ferritin. Haemoglobin does not tell the whole story.

Audrey's story

When she first came to see me, Audrey was a chronically tired 75-year-old. She had been abnormally fatigued for over 30 years, with poor memory and concentration and was 'always cold'. Her GP had described her symptoms as having 'no real cause' except self-inflicted anxiety.

I requested blood tests, which included a thyroid profile consisting of free T4 (thyroxine), free T3 and TSH (thyroid stimulating hormone); all the results were well within the normal ranges. I also requested a ferritin check, which showed an abnormally high level at 430 micrograms/litre (normal range 15-150). Such a high level suggested borderline haemochromatosis.

I also requested an adrenal stress profile, measuring the levels of cortisol and DHEA in her saliva. These results showed a normal cortisol status but a very low DHEA level.

So Audrey's symptoms and test results suggested that she was suffering from iron overload, which had perhaps commenced after her menopause began (at the age of 45) and her periods stopped. The iron loss with periods can protect women from haemochromatosis up to their menopause.

Audrey's treatment for haemochromatosis

The conventional medical treatment for iron overload is bloodletting (phlebotomy). This involves removing blood from the patient, usually once or twice weekly. Each time around 500 millilitres (1 pint) is removed, until the level of ferritin in the blood has normalised. Such a procedure, which although effective is not always popular with patients, is normally prescribed when the ferritin level is in excess of 1000 micrograms/litre. Given Audre's level (430 micrograms), a gentler approach was possible.

I therefore advised Audrey to follow a more nutritional treatment approach. This involved avoiding iron-rich foods coupled with taking supplementary zinc and copper. These two minerals are known to compete with iron absorption at gut level. I have found that the combination of iron avoidance and zinc and copper supplements can be effective in reducing iron overload. Regrettably, with levels in excess of 1000 micrograms/litre, a course of phlebotomy may have to be considered. I also prescribed a course of DHEA to assist Audrey's adrenal fatigue.

A blood test after three months of treatment showed a 15% fall in Audrey's ferritin. This matched improvement in her symptoms (vitality, optimism and mood), which tended to confirm that the long-term iron overload was Audrey's chief problem.

I have recommended that an annual blood test to measure her ferritin status would be advisable, together with a low dosage maintenance routine, taking DHEA, copper and zinc supplements and avoiding iron-rich foods to maintain Audrey's renewed vigour in spite of her age.

Syndrome X

I have described how 'syndrome X' often contributes to the symptoms of CFS, and how it may be diagnosed, earlier in the book (see pages 67 and 135). The condition is variously called 'syndrome X', the 'metabolic syndrome' or 'insulin resistance', but to avoid confusion and duplication I shall refer to it simply as syndrome X. It is refreshingly unusual that this syndrome was not named the 'Reaven syndrome' after Dr Gerald Reaven, who 'discovered' it around 20 years ago. He observed that he was seeing many patients with the same characteristic pattern of symptoms. These symptoms had previously been described as 'pre-diabetes'. The symptoms also very closely matched the accepted risk-factors for heart disease, these being:

1. Obesity
2. Raised blood pressure
3. Raised blood insulin (insulin resistance)
4. Raised blood sugar
5. Raised blood fat (triglycerides)
6. Tendency to low HDL cholesterol ('good' cholesterol)
7. Tendency to high LDL cholesterol ('bad' cholesterol).

With the modern medical tendency to name everything and perhaps to streamline diagnosis and subsequent treatment, Reaven termed this frequently seen grouping of symptoms as syndrome X (or 'Syn.X').

Causes of syndrome X

The chief causes have been described as follows:

1. A family history of heart disease
2. A family history of diabetes
3. Insufficient exercise
4. Cigarette smoking
5. High-sugar and high-carbohydrate diet
6. Excessive weight.

You may be confused to notice the contradictory symptoms of raised blood insulin and raised blood sugar. The obvious question is, if insulin is prescribed for the treatment of diabetes (raised blood sugar), how can raised blood sugar and excessive blood insulin be present at the same time? The answer to this paradox lies in the earlier name for syndrome X – 'pre-diabetes'. Syndrome X, or 'insulin resistance', describes a metabolic imbalance that precedes the full symptoms of type II diabetes. In this state, the cells cease to respond effectively to insulin, resulting in more and more insulin being secreted in an attempt to control the raised blood sugar level.

It is not difficult to identify a common theme that runs through all the syndrome X cluster of symptoms. That is, excessive weight. It is rare to see a person with type II diabetes who is a normal weight. Similarly, with syndrome X patients, an acceptable weight is very unusual. Looking again at the typical metabolic problems that fit the syndrome X description – namely, high blood fats, high blood sugar, high blood pressure, high bad cholesterol and high blood insulin – it is obvious that weight loss is the logical first treatment step.

Geoff's story

When he first came to see me, Geoff was a very tired, overweight IT consultant with a history of high blood pressure and raised blood fats. He fitted many of the diagnostic requirements for syndrome X. I requested the 'metabolic syndrome profile', for Geoff. This was carried out by the Doctors Laboratory in central London, and included the following blood tests:

Triglycerides
Cholesterol
HDL cholesterol

LDL cholesterol

C. reactive protein (CRP)

Insulin

Hb AIC (blood sugar status)

Adiponectin

Hs. CRP.

The results confirmed a diagnosis of syndrome X. In addition, Geoff's weight, at 17.8 stone (246 pounds or 112 kilograms), was excessive and his blood pressure was too high. Geoff was also a heavy smoker (25–30 cigarettes daily). He claimed he was 'too busy to exercise'.

To describe his diet as 'inappropriate' would be an understatement. It included 20-25 strong coffees with sugar each day, plus around 50 units of alcohol each week in addition to a 'hearty' breakfast (usually fried), a sandwich lunch and a cooked evening meal. His work ensured that he was desk-bound and he admitted to using one desk drawer for his 'snack-reserve'; this 'reserve' consisted of crisps, chocolate bars and packets of biscuits. He drove 40–50 miles each day, through busy commuter traffic, and relieved his boredom (and probably his blood sugar imbalance) with regular travel snacks. He had trained his wife to top up his car and another snack reserve in a kitchen cupboard, with his favourite snacks. Although he had two large dogs, his wife was the dog-walker in the family.

When I started practising in the mid-1960s, a patient of 18–20 stone (252–280 pounds or 114–127 kilograms) appeared huge to me and very obviously overweight. Regrettably, with around 50% of the population now overweight, we tend not to notice how big people have become, and a 20-stone person does not appear to be particularly massive. To quote the USA overweight figures, in the mid-1960s, 13% of Americans were obese and around 45% were overweight. By the mid 1990s the figures were 22% obese and a massive 55% were overweight.

There is mounting evidence to confirm the links between excessive weight and high blood fats, high blood pressure and high blood sugar. So, what can be done? Geoff presented a typical set of symptoms and test results for syndrome X. The only clue missing was the absence of any heart or diabetic conditions in his family. (Significantly, his dogs were both overweight and the largest suffered from hypothyroidism.)

Geoff's diet for syndrome X

Geoff needed to lose around 4 stone (56 pounds or 25 kilograms) in weight and achieve improvements in his blood chemistry. I have seen syndrome X patients who have accomplished improvements in all their health problems, simply with weight loss. Excessive weight is fundamental to syndrome X. This particularly applies when the extra weight is around the waist – what is known as 'apple-shaped'.

I advised Geoff seriously to reduce his carbohydrate snacks, cigarettes, coffee and alcohol. I usually prefer to prescribe a diet sheet to patients in preference to verbal advice and I provided Geoff with a copy of my low-carbohydrate diet (see page 149). I also prescribed a supplement programme that included the following vitamins, minerals and proteins:

Vitamins	Minerals	Other
Vitamin B complex	Chromium	Bioflavonoids
Vitamin E	Selenium	Omega-3
Vitamin C	Zinc	Pycnagenol
Vitamin B-12 (high dosage)	Magnesium	Co-enzyme Q-10
Vitamin A	Manganese	
Vitamin D	Potassium	

Many of the above are available within complexes; this can reduce the daily tablet count.

Geoff's exercise programme

Correct exercise is an essential component of any treatment plan for syndrome X. Insulin and glucose levels tend to decrease with exercise. Research has shown that the benefits of exercise can last for two or three days. Insulin efficiency can be prolonged for up to a week after exercise, if the person is in shape and the exercise is regular.

I advised Geoff to do more walking. In addition, he bought a mountain bike for short journeys and also found time to swim twice weekly. Much to his wife's delight, he agreed to do the evening dog walks.

In his excellent book, *Syndrome X*, Gerald Reaven recommended the following simple activities:

Use stairs instead of lifts and elevators

Wash your own car

Mow your own lawn

Walk the dog

Park further from the office and walk in to work

Go dancing and watch less TV

Make an effort to operate the TV without the remote

Try bowling.

Whole-body exercising is usually more beneficial than work-outs on gym equipment. Walking, swimming and cycling are obvious, safe and effective choices.

Geoff's response to treatment

Geoff made progress over a four-month period. His blood fats, sugar control, weight and blood pressure all began to move to normal ranges. He was able gradually to reduce his supplements to a long-term maintenance schedule.

Syndrome X is usually a result of life-style faults and effective treatment needs to include fundamental changes in a person's activities, habits and diet. Fortunately, the symptom improvements achieved motivate many people to maintain a healthier lifestyle.

It is important to have an annual review as a routine; this should include blood testing, weight and blood pressure measurement. If you slip back into a 'couch-potato' life-style, insulin resistance and the symptoms of syndrome X can return.

Diabetes

You may be puzzled to read a case history on type I diabetes included in a book dealing with fatigue, as it is generally assumed that diabetes is efficiently diagnosed and successfully treated within mainstream medicine. This assumption would, however, be false. Perhaps a few statistics will be appropriate. In the UK, there are more than three million diabetics (type I and type II), with approximately 35,000 deaths each year. Diabetes is now the fourth leading cause of death in the UK, only exceeded by cancer, heart disease and the effects of medical treatment. Furthermore, a recent research survey found that up to 35% of insulin-dependent type I diabetics had poorly monitored and badly controlled blood sugar levels.

Diabetes is noted for its wide range of serious complications. These include damage to blood vessels in the eyes, legs, kidneys, brain and heart. Unfortunately, it is often only diagnosed when the symptoms of the complications arise. Once it has been diagnosed, poor control of blood sugar levels make these complications continue to be a risk. Fatigue is a complication that is not so widely recognised.

Matthew's story

Diabetics are often tired. Matthew, a car salesman aged 52 years, with a 20-year history of type I diabetes, complained of fatigue and depression. (As described in chapter 2 (see page 69), type I diabetes is much the less common of the two types; sufferers are usually insulin dependent.) His diabetes had developed shortly after a very stressful divorce.

Matthew considered himself to be 'unnaturally fatigued'. This opinion resulted chiefly from comparing his levels of activity and energy with those of friends and colleagues. He, along with many people, had always assumed that his insulin injections, four times each day, should control his blood sugar, as happens naturally in people without diabetes. Unfortunately, such was his reliance on the injections that he very rarely bothered to check his blood sugar. He only used his glucometer when he suspected an incipient 'hypo' (dangerous drop in blood sugar), which happened two or three times each week.

There are two principal reasons for the unnatural fatigue suffered by insulin-dependent diabetics.

Reason 1: When the blood sugar level falls below 3.0 mmol/l symptoms are likely, potentially leading to a 'hypo', when the sufferer may eventually lose consciousness and have epilepsy-type symptoms. Regrettably, a blood 'hypo' can result in mental and physical after-effects and lethargy for several days.

Reason 2: High levels of blood sugar (that is, in excess of 12-15 mmol/l) can cause excessive thirst and severe restlessness at night. An additional, very distressing symptom is bladder frequency, which will lead to hourly or two-hourly visits to the toilet and consequently severe insomnia. I have spoken to diabetics who are awakened with bladder frequency six to eight times throughout a single night. Understandably, this is stressful, embarrassing and potentially exhausting.

Matthew experienced 'hypos' approximately twice each month and was disturbed virtually nightly, with bladder frequency.

Matthew's treatment

My first priority with Matthew was to make him aware that *all* carbohydrates convert to glucose, and the current medical advice to follow a low-fat and high-complex carbohydrate diet is not ideal. The colour of the bread, cereal, pasta and rice is irrelevant. White and stone-ground brown bread are both carbohydrates, and they both raise blood sugar levels and require insulin to be processed.

Unfortunately, a high-protein diet that has been advocated as ideal for diabetes, in fact also elevates blood insulin, which is not a good idea. The only food group with very little effect on insulin is fat.

Diabetics are currently encouraged to think of fruit sugar (fructose) as a healthy alternative to glucose; this advice can also present problems. **Fructose** is the sweetest of the 'simple' sugars; it is found in fruit, honey and some vegetables. It is recommended because it does not have a significant effect on blood sugar levels and does not require insulin, but this is because it is taken up immediately by the liver where it is rapidly converted into triglycerides – the type of fat that is high risk for heart disease. Unfortunately fructose consumption has increased greatly in the past 20 years, largely as a result of food manufacturers using 'high fructose corn syrup' (HFCS) as a sweetener, which is 55% fructose and 45% glucose.

A recent survey showed that countries that have a high percentage of HFCS in foods and drinks had a 20% higher prevalence of diabetes than countries that did not use HFCS. It seems likely that the human metabolism has not sufficiently evolved to deal with the excessive consumption of fructose contained in HFCS as 'hidden' sugar. In the United States up to 40% of sweeteners are HFCS. Fructose is a risk factor for insulin resistance and type II diabetes, obesity, high blood pressure, heart disease and raised blood triglycerides, as well as many other health problems.

Matthew's diet

Given that carbohydrates in general, and high fructose corn syrup in particular, are problematic for diabetics, you will understand why I redesigned Matthew's diet with the following food group proportions:

Carbohydrates – dietary calories 10%: cereals, sugar, fruit and vegetables etc

Proteins – dietary calories 30%: meat, fish, vegetables, eggs etc

Fat – dietary calories 60%: meat, oils, fish, vegetables, nuts etc.

To fulfil these percentages I advised Matthew to follow my low-carbohydrate diet, described on page 149.

Blood sugar control

Matthew's blood glucose was on a yo-yo schedule, largely as a result of his very casual approach to balancing his diet with his insulin dosages. Treatment for diabetes, especially for type I, requires discipline and self-control. It was clear that his very high night-time glucose levels and his occasional 'hypos' were the chief reasons for his continuing fatigue. The stress resulting from Matthew's disturbed nights, with his wife frequently moving into the spare bedroom, was also contributing to his general depression and fatigue.

Glucometer use

Modern glucose checking with the use of a glucometer is so easy. A simple finger prick with a tiny drop of blood provides the patient's blood glucose level in three to four seconds. Glucometers are easily obtainable and only cost around £12-£15.

The ideal normal range for Matthew's blood sugar level was 4-9 mmol/l. Diabetic nurses have an adage which states, 'under four, on the floor'. This interprets as, if the patient's blood glucose is less than 4 mmol/l, then lie him/her down as quickly as possible, before he/she falls down. The upper limit for a diabetic's recommended range is controversial. I have found that, if possible, it is best to avoid a level in double figures. Many insulin-dependent diabetics see a raised blood sugar as safer than low level as hypos can be very distressing, with bladder incontinence, nausea, tongue-biting and even complete unconsciousness. The diabetic's dread of them is understandable. Nevertheless, frequent nocturnal high levels can be exhausting as a consequence of the bladder frequency and chronic insomnia.

I therefore advised Matthew to check his blood glucose level on rising, on retiring and just before each of his three main meals. He admitted to finding this schedule a little daunting. However, the concept of adjusting his insulin dosage to his next meal made sense and over a period of three to four weeks his sleep settled into an improved pattern. He began to feel in control of his diabetes and the blood testing on retiring and waking provided a guideline to insulin use at night. For the initial three to four weeks he also checked his blood glucose whenever he awakened during the night. This also assisted his control.

His fatigue and depression improved and he was then able to develop a less frequent blood check programme, which he found reassuring but essential. He was now in control of his diabetes, which ensured it was no longer causing symptoms, and he willingly followed his treatment guidelines.

Supplements to support blood sugar control

Some years ago I formulated a supplement, the Glycaemic Complex™, for the nutritional support of blood sugar control in type I and type II diabetes. This is produced by Nutri Advanced Ltd, a company based in Derbyshire which has provided supplements for practitioners for more than 30 years. It contains:

Vitamin A (as beta carotene)	Selenium
Vitamin A (as retinyl acetate)	Magnesium
Vitamin B-1	Manganese
Vitamin B-2	Copper
Vitamin B-3	Calcium
Vitamin B-6	Zinc
Vitamin B-12	Potassium
Vitamin E	Alpha-lipoic acid
Folate	Quercetin
Inositol	Pycnogenol
Pantothenic acid	Grape seed extract
Biotin	Ground cinnamon bark
Chromium	Green tea leaf.

Prior to the complex being available I was often obliged to prescribe 10-12 capsules and tablets for my diabetic patients, hence the value of a complex of nutrients in one formula.

Less common causes of CFS – diagnosis and treatment

Drug side-effects

Polypharmacy is a word now used to describe the taking of lots of different prescription pills and medicines. The annual number of prescriptions average around 20 per person in the UK. This number has doubled in 10 years. It is now quite usual to see patients over 65 years taking eight to 12 different types of medication daily. The potential to suffer side-effects of course increases with the number of prescriptions.

Very little research is being done to learn about the effects of polypharmacy. Understandably, drug manufacturers do not offer large budgets to study side-effects. This particularly applies to side-effects from drug combinations (drug interactions).

The most frequently experienced side-effect is fatigue. This includes mental fatigue, which is usually expressed as poor memory and concentration. The 'yellow card scheme', which is run by the Medicines and Healthcare Products Regulatory Agency (MHRA), allows you to report suspected side-effects (see https://yellowcard.mhra.gov.uk/ for further details). (To find out what side-effects a drug may cause, consult the *British National Formulary* or *BNF*, which the NHS supplies to all its doctors.)

Treatment

If you consider that your CFS may be caused by, or worsened by, drug side-effects, online research and a discussion with your GP are the two obvious lines of inquiry.

Chronic infections and CFS

Epstein-Barr virus (EBV)

The most serious form of EBV is known as 'infectious mononucleosis' or 'glandular fever' (the 'kissing disease'). The symptoms of most of the EBV infections are similar to those of a cold or viral illness. Infectious mononucleosis may be passed among teenagers and young adults by kissing or intimate contact. The major symptom is extreme fatigue, and full convalescence can take many weeks.

Blood tests to detect antibodies to EBV are usually requested to confirm mononucleosis. It has been estimated that in the US population, nearly 95% of all adults have had EBV infections.

Cytomegalovirus (CMV) or herpes virus

Many people infected with CMV do not show symptoms. It can cause serious symptoms in pregnant women (including miscarriage and infant death) and those whose immune system has been weakened (AIDS, for example), potentially leading to blindness or even death. The virus can remain dormant in various tissues for a person's whole lifetime. Diagnosis can be made by blood testing.

CMV – treatment

In recent years the amino acid (protein) lysine has acquired a reputation for successfully treating the herpes virus. However, it may also be necessary to address problems with immune-system efficiency, including thyroid and adrenal health.

Chronic hepatitis

Hepatitis is inflammation of the liver from any cause. Choosing the right tests for it is therefore a complex exercise. There are various profiles, antibodies and genotypes that may be checked. Acute hepatitis is usually caused by a virus, of which there are five types – A, B, C, D and E. Hepatitis can also result from viral infections, such as mononucleosis, yellow fever and cytomegalovirus.

Chronic hepatitis can develop gradually over a period of years. It may worsen into cirrhosis of the liver and even liver cancer. There are many causes of hepatitis, including alcoholism, drug side-effects, poor hygiene and drug addicts sharing needles.

Chronic hepatitis – treatment

Treatment for hepatitis will depend on its cause(s) and whether it is the acute or chronic variety. The chief herbal remedy is milk thistle (silybum marianum). Raw liver (bovine) glandulars can also help.

Supplements of special value include vitamin B-12, vitamin C and vitamin A; the amino acids L.carnitine, glutathione and L-cysteine; and co-enzyme Q-10, essential fatty acids and garlic.

Acupuncture is also a useful therapy.

Multiple chemical sensitivity syndrome (MCSS)

MCSS is a very common syndrome contributing to CFS (see page 80). Perhaps with MCSS, the priority is not treatment, but rather identifying and, where possible, eliminating the culprits in your own environment. Certainly, personal research is worthwhile, as there may be several domestic, workspace and other chemical sensitivity sources in your daily environment that are contributing to your low state of vitality. There are many that are well defined and obvious; you could start to reduce or avoid your contact with drugs, alcohol, caffeine, nicotine, car exhausts and food additives.

Low-frequency sound

The effect of low-frequency sound is an interesting and controversial subject that we are going to be made more aware of in the near future (see page 80). The only really effective treatment is to avoid wind farms and move house. It must be in your best interest to be aware of plans to erect giant wind farms in your neighbourhood. There are now more than 4,000 wind turbines in the UK and many are double the size of those erected 15 years ago.

Aero-toxic syndrome

Air contamination ('fume events') can cause symptoms on regular or prolonged flights. The symptoms result from air in the passenger cabin originating from the engines and being contaminated with oil fumes, additives and the products of oil decomposition. Aero-toxic syndrome is a well-known phenomenon, so much so that the latest aircraft designs are *not* using air from the engines in the passenger cabins.

As is so often the case with any form of toxaemia, sensitivity or pollution, fatigue is the main symptom that arises.

Toxic metals

Aside from mercury amalgam in teeth, the chief sources of toxic metal poisoning are: industrial; pesticides and other sprays; drugs; dietary sources. A detailed listing can be found on page 81.

Diagnosis of metal toxicity involves either blood testing or hair mineral analysis. Testing can also be done on urine and sweat. There are advantages and disadvantages to both main methods of testing.

Hair mineral analysis

The chief advantage of hair-mineral analysis is its low cost (around £95 in the UK). The following **minerals** may be tested:

Calcium	Copper	Manganese	Selenium
Chromium	Iron	Phosphorus	Sodium
Cobalt	Magnesium	Potassium	Zinc

And the following **toxic metals**:

Aluminium	Lead
Arsenic (a 'trace' metal)	Mercury
Cadmium	Nickel.

The chief disadvantage of hair analysis is the need for the hair sample to be free from bleach, highlights, 'perms' and tinting. Colourings, shampoos and conditioners are acceptable, but the chemicals contained in them must be known and listed. Another obvious problem with hair analysis is the need for adequate hair (around 2 grams).

Blood mineral screen (+ Heavy metals)

The blood mineral profile is included in the Doctors Laboratory laboratory guide as the 'Trace Metal (blood) Profile'. The metals in this profile are listed as:

Aluminium	Copper	Magnesium	Zinc
Calcium	Iron	Manganese	
Chromium	Lead	Mercury	

The main advantage of blood over hair mineral analysis is the ease with which patients can be prepared (a short fast with no worries about the state of their hair) and the sample taken. Blood testing is also seen as a more accurate and less controversial method. The main disadvantage is the relatively high cost (£190 in the UK) of the blood profile. You will also have observed that the blood profile only includes 11 minerals while hair analysis measures 18. Both tests are carried out by the Doctors Laboratory in central London.

Toxic metals – treatment
The testing, diagnosis and treatment of toxic metal poisoning is a very specialised area of health care.

Omega-3 and omega-6 deficiency
Omega-3 and omega-6 are polyunsaturated fatty acids, which the body needs but cannot manufacture itself. Hormones with an omega-3 base have a tendency to reduce inflammation and those with an omega-6 base increase it. There is an element of competition between omega-3 and omega-6 in forming the membranes of our cells. The ratio of the omegas in our cell membranes is seen to have an influence on inflammatory conditions, such as heart disease, rheumatoid arthritis, Crohn's disease, colitis, asthma, dysmenorrhoea, coronary artery disease and migraines. Consequently, the types of fat that we eat, in particular the omega-3 fatty acids, can make a difference to inflammatory and immune system problems.

I cannot resist another quotation from Robert Atkins's excellent book (see Further reading, page 247), in which he writes: 'Our biggest problem is that during the course of the 20th century, we have eaten too many omega-6 fats – safflower, sunflower and corn oil – and have virtually eliminated foods high in the omega-3s, such as flaxseed oil and cold-water fish.'

Unfortunately, one of the chief sources of omega-6 is evening primrose oil; it is consumed in huge quantities because it is reputed to an effective treatment for pre-menstrual syndrome (PMS). The modern western diet is characteristically high in omega-6 fatty acids, low in omega-3 fatty acids and high in sugar. It is therefore pro-inflammatory.

The current ratio of omega-6 to omega-3 in western nations is around 15 to 1. Many specialists and researchers argue that an ideal ratio should be 2 to 1. This unfortunately is not easy to achieve with a diet rich in omega-6-rich foods. Supplementation of omega-3 is feasible, but many of us lack direction or dosage guidance. Your practitioner should be able to advise what is right specifically for you.

Omega-3 and omega-6 – diagnosis and treatment

The test of choice to assess our omega-3 to omega-6 ratio is called the 'essential red cell fatty acids omega-3/omega-6' test. I request this through the Doctors Laboratory in central London. A recommendation for the most appropriate supplementation to achieve the optimal ratio is provided with each set of results. I find such testing reduces or even eliminates the guesswork that so often is the case in recommending supplements. Follow-up testing as well as improvement in symptoms can accurately point to possible future treatment requirements (see page 119).

Histamine intolerance (HIT)

At the moment the NHS does not finance laboratory testing for HIT. Perhaps this is just as well, as very few laboratories offer the two essential tests. These measure diamine oxidase (DAO), an enzyme that metabolises histamine, and blood histamine itself. Although many laboratories will carry out histamine checks, lack of demand causes lack of interest in DAO testing. Histamine intolerance is indicated by a low DAO level and a high blood histamine. Although DAO can be purchased and taken as a supplementary enzyme tablet, it is costly and is thought to offer only transient symptom relief.

Fructose, lactose and histamine intolerances are often tested together. This type of testing is more widespread in German and Austrian clinics, but remains quite rare in the UK. For those readers with an interest in HIT, Genny Masterman's book, *What HIT Me? Living with Histamine Intolerance*, is well worth reading (see Further reading, page 250).

Air pollution

Not surprisingly, the chief cause of urban air pollution in the UK is traffic fumes. I recently spoke to one of my patients whose eight-year-old daughter developed asthma six months after the family moved into the centre of a town. The road immediately outside the house was full of queuing cars most of the day. Within 12 months they had moved again to the outskirts of the town, with much less traffic. The daughter's asthma had virtually cleared, four months after the move.

Unfortunately, there are many households living adjacent to heavy traffic. This is one of the common environmental causes of ill health, including CFS, to which there is no immediate answer for many people. However, an awareness of the possible causes of symptoms based on a little detective work must be worthwhile. It is not unusual for CFS sufferers to feel noticeably more vital when living away from their home or on holiday. Such a transition should prompt an investigation into possible environmental symptoms that may be location-specific and treatable.

Obviously domestic and work stress may play a part in such a scenario and may therefore also need to be considered.

The next step

When I discuss my patients' health problems with them, including their symptoms, past treatments and their general health history, I am often obliged to remind them that people have an annoying habit of being 'different'. I am sure that medical doctors, naturopaths and practitioners of the many various therapies available, would welcome a certain patient standardisation. If, when a patient mentioned symptoms, we knew precisely what they meant, what their symptom severity was and the effects on their health, it would greatly assist the accuracy and success of any diagnosis and treatment.

Although, for ease of diagnosis, symptoms are often grouped into syndromes, a symptom is a subjective experience that can only be described and defined by the patient. It may surprise you to learn that a good medical dictionary will describe in excess of 1,100 symptom complexes or syndromes, usually named simply to describe the appearance of the symptoms or the 'inventor' of the syndrome. These include such beauties as:

Alice-in-Wonderland syndrome
Blackfan-diamond syndrome
Chinese restaurant syndrome
Happy puppet syndrome
Holiday heart syndrome
Morning glory syndrome

One-and-a-half syndrome

Prune belly syndrome

Social breakdown syndrome

Tired housewife syndrome

Whistling face syndrome

And last but certainly not least, hyperornithinemia-hyperammonemia-
homocitrullinuria syndrome.

I see many patients whose symptoms have never been diagnosed as an illness, let alone a syndrome. They often express a longing to be given a name for their condition. Perhaps in the absence of a title to describe their ill-health, they are afraid to be termed 'neurotic' and prescribed a placebo remedy to simply provide symptom relief.

The great variations in symptoms tend to make diagnosis and treatment selection a challenge for any practitioner. Although we all rely on the previous experience of treating similar cases, sometimes definitive test results can show the way to a fairly exact and objective diagnostic decision.

Treatment selection

Public confidence in mainstream medicine is at an all-time low. We are frequently reminded that the NHS is Europe's largest employer, but size does not unfortunately guarantee excellence. In the UK, patients are very lucky if they have more than a 10-minute interview with their general practitioner (GP) and for most of this time their GP will be staring at their computer screen. Patients are often advised to 'bring in' a maximum of three symptoms for discussion. In common with many of my colleagues, I allow a 60-minute appointment for new patients and 30 minutes for follow-up appointments. Even with such a time allowance, I frequently run late!

Practitioner selection

For the exhausted CFS patient seeking help, there are two priority decisions. These are the selection of a therapy and the selection of a therapist. Although one cannot expect to receive guarantees for treatment results from any practitioner, an outline of procedure and treatment, time-scale and costs, should not be too much to expect.

A consultation with any professional person is by definition a meeting or an interview; this being based on known facts. I see the consultation as a time for the patient and the practitioner to ask questions. I never take offence when a patient asks me, 'Do you treat my type of health problem?' The modern trend, prior to booking an appointment, and again prior to a face-to-face meeting, is to exchange emails. However, I know some colleagues who strongly object to discussing health problems over the internet with people they have not met. Some years ago I was initially resentful at the over familiarity so often expressed online. However, emails are here to stay and I now wonder how we managed without them. I live in rural France and contact with the UK by post is costly and sometimes very slow. To send an email, and at times receive a response within an hour, can be very helpful and time-saving. Probably half my new patients' appointments are currently made via the internet, very often following an interchange of emails. However, I always insist on a face-to-face meeting for the patient's initial consultation. I sometimes agree to telephone for follow-up appointments, if patients live far away or are disabled.

So, those of you who are uncertain just who to consult with your CFS symptoms, do not be afraid to email various practitioners and seek information on their diagnostic and treatment methods and their experience of treating your type of problem. Should their reply state that they cannot comment or advise you prior to seeing you, then try elsewhere. An informative, reassuring email can be composed in a few minutes. This type of information-gathering is essential in my case, as many potential patients are unfamiliar with naturopathic practice and quite rightly wish to know more. Many think naturopathic treatment involves cold bathing, enemas and fasting. In fact, modern naturopathic practice embraces nutritional medicine, supplement use and many ancillary alternative therapies.

Visiting your GP

Those readers who are suffering from CFS will very likely have already consulted their GP. Unfortunately, the search for a diagnosis and treatment via the NHS is rarely a satisfactory journey, though no doubt there are CFS patients who have found the experience rewarding and worthwhile. Not surprisingly, I rarely meet such patients, being usually the second or third choice of practitioner after disappointing visits to GPs and consultants.

The most common diagnosis offered by GPs for CFS is stress or depression and the usual treatment offered is anti-depressants.

In spite of the many differences in approach between mainstream and alternative medicine, there is also some common ground. This can be seen chiefly in blood test selection. Probably around 50% of the blood test results that I see are tests requested and made available through my patients' GPs. Loss of good will and co-operation between non-medical and medical practitioners always leads to extra stress and expense for the patient.

When discussing blood test requirements with my patients, I always mention that the only difference between NHS and private laboratory testing is that, when I request certain tests, the patient has to pay. A routine fatigue profile, including vitamin B-12, ferritin and a thyroid profile, would privately cost around £100. I have an account with the Doctors Laboratory in Wimpole Street, London, so no charge is made for phlebotomy (sample taking). However, I always receive the laboratory test results on the following day by email. The other obvious advantage, aside from the speed of private testing as opposed to NHS testing, is that of test selection. Modern laboratories often have a 2000+ test 'menu', so the correct choice of tests is vital.

NHS laboratories are currently cost-cutting, making some test results hard to obtain, As I have described earlier in the book, NHS laboratories will often not perform a requested free T4 (thyroxine) test if the result of a TSH (thyroid stimulating hormone) test is normal. Likewise, the test for ferritin (iron stores) is often a 'special request test' and is not carried out when the patient has 'normal' haemoglobin. Meanwhile, the new test for vitamin B-12, known as 'active B-12', is not yet available in NHS laboratories. I have spoken to GPs who have experienced concern and annoyance that tests that they have requested have been crossed out by laboratory staff, usually as a result of a cost-cutting policy.

In spite of such problems, I still see many patients whose GPs request their various blood tests on a regular basis and they let me have copies of the results. For patients to be caught between two, often conflicting, systems of medicine can sometimes lead to additional stress and uncertainty. I never mind providing reports and supplement details to patients, at the request of their GPs.

I regularly make use of the services of specialised private laboratories, examples being Biolab, Genova, the Doctors Laboratory and Acumen. Such laboratories offer specific, and often unique, functional tests that are not usually part of the NHS remit. Nonetheless, the vast majority of the required tests for CFS patients are available through the NHS via a co-operative GP.

You may wonder, just why is a naturopath not only praising, but recommending medical methods to assist CFS diagnosis. Perhaps the answer lies in the answer to the question, 'Who are my typical patients?' My typical patients are exhausted people, often lacking in self-confidence, in finance and in patience. I have seen CFS patients who have suffered from their symptoms for over 20 years, have subsequently parted from their husband or wife, lost their job and career prospects, and are virtually reclusive drop-outs. Such people become vulnerable to therapies or therapists who offer solutions at a price. I have spoken to patients who have invested more than £10,000 in private medical tests and treatment programmes, this often without any real health improvement.

Although I have criticised the NHS approach frequently in this book, I am the first to admit that medical practitioners usually display a more dependable code of ethics and clinical efficiency than many private therapists.

Overall summary

So I do hope that this book has offered readers food for thought. (I am sorry, but I could not resist that maxim.) Whatever diagnostic pathway you as a patient may choose to follow, look at the obvious before the exotic. Simple, iron-deficient anaemia, an under-active thyroid, or vitamin B-12 deficiency, may be major contributors to your fatigue. These may need to be identified and treated before more obscure causes and conditions are addressed. The concept of a 'second opinion' is fundamental to medical thinking, so do not be afraid to look again. Should a doctor or naturopath express resentment that you are looking for another opinion, then you can always remind him or her that the concept is integral to medical ethos.

I have observed one common characteristic shown by CFS patients: the nature of their symptoms serves to ensure that they do not give in easily. I do hope that this resolve applies to all you readers.

Further reading

Alison Adams. *Chronic Fatigue, M.E. and Fibromyalgia – the natural recovery plan*. Published by Watkins Publishing, 2010

Ridha Arem, Dr. *The Thyroid Solution*. Published by Ballantine Books, 2007

Robert Atkins. *Dr Atkins Vita-Nutrient Solution*. Published by Simon and Schuster, 2002

H Atkinson. *Women and Fatigue*. Published by Pocket Books, 1998 (out of print)

Broda Barnes *Hypo-thyroidism: The Unsuspected Illness*. Published by Harper and Row, 1990

F Batmanghelidj. *Your Body's Many Cries For Water*. Published by Tagman, 2008

Jane L Billett and O J Seiden. *5-HTP – The Serotonin Connection*. Published by Prima Health, 2012

Jeffery Bland. *Clinical Nutrition – A Functional Approach*. Published by the Institute for Functional Medicine. (Latest edition, 2012.)

Gerald P Bodey. *Candidiasis*. Published by Raven Press, 1993 (out of print)

Martin Budd. *Low Blood Sugar*. Published by Thorsons, 1983

Martin Budd. *Eat to Beat Low Blood Sugar*. Published by Thorsons, 2009

Martin Budd. *Why Am I So Tired?* Published by Harper Collins, 2000

Martin Budd. *Why Can't I Lose Weight?* Published by Harper Collins, 2002

Frankie Campling and Michael Sharpe. *Chronic Fatigue Syndrome*. Published by Oxford University Press, 2008

Geoffrey Cannon. *Superbug*. Published by Virgin, 1996

Rachel Carson. *Silent Spring*. Published by Penguin, 1962

Peter Cartwright. *Probiotics for Crohn's and Colitis*. Published by Prentice Publishing, 2003

Leon Chaitow. *Postviral Syndrome*. Published by JM Dent and Sons, 1989 (out of print)

Leon Chaitow. *The Raw Materials of Health*. Published by Thorsons, 1989 (out of print)

Jack Challem, Burton Berkson and Melissa Diane Smith. *Syndrome X*. Published by John Wiley & Sons, 2001

Anthony Cichoke Dr. *The Complete Book of Enzyme Therapy*. Published by Avery Publishing, 1998

Greg Critser. *Fat Land*. Published by Allen Lane, 2004 (out of print)

William G Crook. *The Yeast Connection*. Published by Square One Publishing, 2008

Belinda Davies, Damien Downing and Belinda Dawes. *Why ME?* Published by Grafton Books 1989 (out of print)

Stephen Davies, Alan Stewart and Andrew Stanway. *Nutritional Medicine*. Published by Pan Books, 1987 (out of print)

Thomas Royle Dawber. *The Framingham Study*. Published by Harvard University Press

Rob Dunn. *The Wild Life of Our Bodies*. Published by Harper, 2011

Barry Durrant-Peatfield. *Your Thyroid and How to Keep it Healthy*. Published by Hammersmith Press, 2006

Micheal Eades and Mary Eades. *Protein Power*. Published by Thorsons, 2011

Further Reading

Udo Erasmus. *Fats that Heal. Fats that Kill*. Published by Alive Books, 1993

Joe Fitzgibbon. *Feeling Tired All The Time*. Published by Gill and Macmillan, 2001 (out of print)

Gillian Ford and Susan Silva. *Listening to Your Hormones*. Published by Prima Publishing, 1997

Carlton Fredericks and H Goodman. *Low Blood Sugar and You*. Published by Perigee, 1994 (out of print)

Alex Gazzola. *Coeliac Disease*. Published by Sheldon Press, 2011

Ben Goldacre. *Bad Science*. Published by Fourth Estate, 2009

Ben Goldacre. *Bad Pharma*. Published by Fourth Estate, 2012

Barry Groves. *Eat Fat, Get Thin*. Published by Vermillion, 2000

Barry Groves. *Trick and Treat*. Published by Hammersmith Press, 2008

Barry Groves. *Natural Health and Weight Loss*. Published by Hammersmith Press, 2007

Morland Hammitt and Teri Rumpf. *The Sjögren's Syndrome*. Published by New Harbinger Publishing, 2003

Collette Harris and Adam Carey. *PCOS – a woman's guide to dealing with polycystic ovary syndrome*. Published by Thorsons, 2011

Diana Holmes. *Tears Behind Closed Doors*. Published by Avon Books, 2002 (out of print)

Martyn Hooper. *Pernicious Anaemia – the forgotten disease*. Published by Hammersmith Health Books, 2012

Chris Jenner. *Fibromyalgia and Myofascial Pain Syndrome*. Published by How to Books, 2011

David S Jones. *Textbook of Functional Medicine*. Published by the Institute for Functional Medicine, 2010 (out of print)

Mohammed Kalimi and William Regelson. *The Biologic Role of Dehydroepiandrosterone*. Published by Walter de Gruyter, 1990 (out of print)

L Kennedy and A Basu. *Problem Solving in Endocrinology and Metabolism*. Published by Clinical Publishing, 2006

Anne MacIntyre Dr. *ME Post Viral Fatigue Syndrome*. Published by Unwin Paperbacks, 1989 (out of print)

Gale Maleskey and Mary Kittel. *The Hormone Connection*. Published by Prevention, 2003 (out of print)

Genny Masterman. *What HIT Me? Living with Histamine Intolerance*. Published by Genny Masterman, 2011

Jeffrey C May. *My House is Killing Me*. Published by John Hopkins University Press, 2001

Kilmer S McCully. *The Homocysteine Revolution*. Published by Keats Publishing, 1999

Erik Millstone. *Lead and Public Health: the dangers for childrten*. Published by Earthscan, 1997 (out of print)

Michael Moss. *Salt, Sugar, Fat*. Published by Whallen, 2013

Sarah Myhill. *Diagnosing and Treating Chronic Fatigue Syndrome*. Published by Hammersmith Health Books, 2014

Roger Newman-Turner. *Naturopathic Medicine*. Published by Health Advisory, 2000 (out of print)

Sally M Pacholok and Jeffrey L Stuart. *Could it be B12?* Published by Quill Driver, 2011

Sue Pemberton and Catherine Berry. *Fighting Fatigue*. Published by Hammersmith Press, 2009

Raymond Perrin. *The Perrin Technique – how to beat CFS/ME*. Published by Hammersmith Press, 2007

Carl Pfeiffer. *Mental and Elemental Nutrients*. Published by Keats Publishers Inc, 1975 (out of print)

J Picazo. *Glucagon*. Published by Kluwer Academic Publishers, 2012

Walter Pierpaoli, William Regelson and Carol Colman. *The Melatonin Miracle*. Published by Simon and Schuster, 1995 (out of print)

Weston Price. *Nutrition and Physical Degeneration*. Published by Price-Pottenger Foundation, 2010

Proceedings of the Oxford Symposiums on Food and Cookery 1983 – 2012. Published by Prospect Books, 1983–2012 (annual)

Basant Puri. *Chronic Fatigue Syndrome*. Published by Hammersmith Press, 2005

Melvin Ramsay. *Postviral Fatigue Syndrome*. Published by Gower Medical, 1986 (out of print)

William J Rea. *Chemical Sensitivity*. Published by CRC Press, 1996 (out of print)

Gerald Reaven. *Syndrome X*. Published by Simon and Schuster, 2001

Paul Robinson. *Recovering with T3*. Published by Paul Robinson, 2011

Ray Sahelian. *Melatonin – Nature's Sleeping Pill*. Published by Be Happier Press, 1995 (out of print)

Eric Schlosser. *Fast Food Nation*. Published by Penguin Books, 2002

Hans Selye Dr. *The Stress of Life*. Published by McGraw-Hill, 1978

David G Smith. *Understanding Myalgic Encephalomyelitis*. Published by Robinson Publishing, 1989

Henry Solomon. *The Exercise Myth*. Published by Harper Collins Ltd, 1985

Paul St Amand and Claudia Craig Marek. *What Your Doctor May Not Tell You About Fibromyalgia*. Published by Grand Central Publishing, 2012

Jacob Teitelbaum. *From Fatigue to Fantastic*. Published by Avery, 2007

Ross Trattler and Shea Trattler. *Better Health Through Natural Healing*. Published by Hinkler Books, 2013

Orian Truss. *The Missing Diagnosis*. Published by Truss, 1985 (out of print)

Erica Verillo and Lauron Gellman. *Chronic Fatigue Syndrome – a treatment guide*. Published by St Martin's Griffen, 1998 (out of print)

Morton Walker. *DMSO*. Published by Avery Publishing Group, 2000

Daniel J Wallace. *The Lupus book*, fifth edition. Published by Oxford University Press, 2012

Michael A Weiner. *Maximum Immunity*. Published by Gateway Books, 1986 (out of print)

Gilbert Welch, Lisa Schwartz and Steve Woloskin. *Overdiagnosed – making people sick in pursuit of health*. Published by Beacon Press, 2012

Melvyn R Werbach. *Nutritional Influences on Illness*. Published by Thorsons, 1996 (out of print)

Manfred Wick, W Pinggera and Peter Lehmann. *Clinical Aspects of Laboratory Iron Metabolism*. Published by Springer Vienna, 2003 (out of print)

Steve Wilkinson. *ME and You*. Published by Thorsons, 1988 (out of print)

Will Wilkoff. *Is My Child Overtired?*. Published by Simon and Schuster, 2001

Roger Williams. *Nutrition Against Disease*. Published by Pitman Publishing, 1981 (out of print)

Roger J Williams. *Biochemical Individuality*. Published by University of Texas Press, 1998

Bee Wilson. *Swindled*. Published by John Murray, 2009

James L Wilson. *Adrenal Fatigue*. Published by Smart Publications, 2002

Celia Wookey. *Myalgic Encephalomyelitis*. Published by Chapman and Hall, 1988 (out of print)

Sam Ziff. *The Toxic Time Bomb*. Published by Thorsons, 1985 (out of print)

Glossary

Achlorhydria: Virtual absence of hydrochloric stomach acid.

Acid:Any substance with a pH less than 7. Acids are sour tasting and corrosive. The balancing compounds are termed alkali (or base).

Active vitamin B-12: A recently developed blood test. Unlike the previous B-12 test which measured the total vitamin B-12, the active test is a more accurate reflection of B-12 status.

Acute: The term used to describe a symptom or condition with a rapid onset, usually of short duration. An acute condition can be severe, such as a fever or pain.

Addison's disease: Severe adrenal insufficiency or failure. Causes can be an auto-immune condition, stress, infection or trauma.

Adenosinediphosphate (ADP): This compound is converted from ATP to supply energy and then recycled back to ATP.

Adenosine monophosphate (AMP) This compound results from excessive energy use and is converted from ADP. AMP represents an energy cul-de-sac and leads to fatigue. AMP recycling can occur but only very slowly.

Adenosinetriphosphate (ATP): A chemical compound that is our energy currency, provided by the mitochondria in cells.

Adrenal glands: Two glands located at the top of each kidney; consisting of two portions, the cortex and medulla. The cortex secretes cortisol (hydrocortisone), cortisone and adrenal androgens. The androgens are precursors of testosterone and the oestrogens. The medulla secretes adrenaline (epinephrine) and nor-adrenaline (norepinephrine).

Adrenalcorticotrophic hormone (ACTH): A hormone secreted by the pituitary gland to stimulate the production of cortisol and other adrenal hormones.

Adrenaline (epinephrine): A hormone produced by the adrenal glands to facilitate sudden physical activity in an emergency and to raise the blood sugar level. Referred to as the 'fight or flight' response.

Adrenal stress profile (Genova Diagnostics): Test to measure the levels of the adrenal hormones DHEA and cortisol, using four saliva samples over a single day.

Aerotoxic stress: Air contamination in aircraft. Symptoms result from the air in the passenger cabin originating from the aircraft engines. The chief symptom is fatigue.

Aetiology: The cause of a disease or disorder.

Aldosterone: A hormone produced by the adrenal cortex. It influences sodium and potassium levels in the cells and blood and greatly influences fluid volume.

Alkali: Any substance with a pH in excess of 7.

Alpha lipoic acid (thioctic acid): An anti-oxidant compound of great value in the treatment of diabetic neuropathy and insulin resistance. Prescribed to prevent brain cell damage in Alzheimer's disease. It also reduces harm to the liver from alcoholism and is prescribed to treat AIDS.

Alzheimer's disease: Progressive brain deterioration characterised by changes in the nerve cells in the brain; the most common cause of dementia. Symptoms can include memory loss, confusion, restlessness, tremor, speech disturbance. Symptoms have been linked with and compared to aluminium and mercury toxicity.

Amino acids: These are the 'building blocks' of proteins. There are 20 different amino acids. The body can make some; others are needed in food ('essential').

Anaemia: A low level of red blood cells/haemoglobin. Causes include a reduction in red cell production, increased red cell destruction and blood loss. Classification is determined by the haemoglobin level and by the red cell size.

There are more than 90 different named anaemias, usually defined by their cause, the commonest being iron-deficient anaemia.

Androgens: The male sex hormones. In males androgens are produced by the testes and the adrenal glands, but in females, only by the adrenal glands.

Anorexia nervosa: Metabolic disorder seen chiefly in young females. Refusal to eat in an attempt to lose weight leading to self-starvation which can cause death. The condition has been linked to zinc deficiency. Symptoms can include fatigue, anaemia, cessation of periods, hypotension, loss of teeth and bone quality, with poor bone density over a period.

Antioxidants: Substances produced either by our metabolism or by dietary supplements that prevent chemical oxidation in the body from occurring too rapidly. They can prevent the build-up of unpaired electrons within the cells.

Anxiety: Fearful state and emotional tension. Many causes including hypoglycaemia, adrenal fatigue, exhaustion, pre-menstrual syndrome, stress, conflict and depression.

Armour thyroid: Natural desiccated thyroid; produced from bovine or porcine sources. Preferred by many over synthetic thyroxine as its use falls between the synthetic thyroxine and the hormone-free glandulars.

Attention-deficit hyperactivity disorder (ADHD): Poor or short-term attention span and impulsiveness inappropriate for a child's age. Can include hyperactivity. Often misdiagnosed and treated incorrectly. Thought by many to be related to blood sugar metabolism, food allergies and excessive antibiotic prescriptions for children.

Autism: A mental disorder characterised by poor communication skills, delusions and a withdrawal from reality. Sufferers are usually totally self-centred and lacking in empathy.

Auto-immune diseases: Disorders in which the immune system mistakenly attacks the body. The precise cause is unknown.

Autonomic nervous system: A part of the nervous system that regulates non-voluntary functions. These include heart muscle, the intestines and the endocrine glands. It sub-divides into the sympathetic and the parasympathetic branches of the nervous system.

Bacteria: Single-cell organisms that are generally beneficial, but harmful usually as a result of human interventions and/or imbalance.

Barnes temperature test: A thyroid function test, devised by Dr Broda Barnes. The test involves measuring the underarm temperature on waking for three consecutive mornings. Low levels can be found in mild hypothyroidism. This basal temperature test was researched in the 1940s and has recently been seen as unreliable as a method to diagnose an underactive thyroid.

Basophils: One of the types of white cell in the blood. Responsible for the secretion of IgE immunoglobulins, which cause the histamine reactions common to allergies and tissue inflammation.

Body mass index (BMI): The recommended weight to height ratio. Calculated by dividing your weight in kilograms by the square of your height in metres (kg/m^2). A healthy BMI is seen as 20–25. Over 25 is judged overweight and 30+ clinically obese.

Bulimia: Alternating binge-eating and self-induced vomiting. Usually seen in young women with a frequent psychiatric component. Symptoms include fatigue, digestive conditions, dehydration, abdominal pain, dental problems, low blood potassium and swollen ankles.

Calorie: The amount of heat required to raise the temperature of one gram of water by 1°C. The total amount of heat available from the full combustion of food is 4.1 kcal per gram from carbohydrates, 4.3 kcal per gram from protein and 9.0 kcal per gram from fat. In nutritional and metabolic studies the kilocalorie is generally abbreviated to calorie, but written with a capital C to indicate that it is the larger unit.

Candidiasis: Chronic overgrowth of the yeast *Candida albicans*. Symptoms can include thrush and leaky gut etc.

Caprylic acid: A short chain fatty acid; its main use is in the treatment of candidiasis.

Carnitine: An amino acid, used to reduce blood fat levels and heart disorders and often referred to as 'the fat burner'. Found mainly in red meat, it requires the co-factors iron and vitamin C to prevent a deficiency. It is an essential component of cellular energy metabolism.

Carpal tunnel syndrome: Compression of the median nerve in the wrist. Symptoms include paraesthesia in the first three fingers, which causes clumsiness. Worse at night. Can lead to muscle wasting. Usually treated with cortico-steroid injections or surgery. Chiefly affects middle-aged women.

Cholesterol: A fat-soluble substance occurring in animal fats, oils and various foods. It is found in the bile, blood, brain, liver, kidneys, adrenal glands and nerves. It is the precursor of the steroid and sex hormones, including cortisol, DHEA, oestrogen and progesterone. It can crystallise in the gall bladder to form gallstones. Incorrectly linked to strokes and heart disorders, only 20% of total cholesterol is dietary, the remaining 80% being produced by the liver.

Chronic: (As distinct from acute) A long-term illness, or symptoms which persist or recur over a lengthy period. It does not imply anything concerning severity.

Cobalamin: Another name for vitamin B-12.

Coeliac disease: Sensitivity to gluten, found in wheat, oats, barley and rye. The small intestine fails efficiently to digest and absorb food. Usually classed as an auto-immune condition. The problem component of gluten is gliadin, a natural protein in grains.

Co-enzyme Q-10 (Ubiquinone): An essential component of energy production in every cell. Statins (anti-cholesterol drugs) inhibit the body's natural ability to make co-enzyme Q-10.

Corticoid: Any of the C21 steroids produced by the adrenal cortex.

Cortisol: A steroid hormone, produced by the adrenal cortex. Functions include glucose metabolism, protein and fat regulation and immune system regulation. It also functions as an anti-inflammatory corticoid.

Cortisone: An anti-inflammatory hormone produced by the adrenal glands. It can be converted into cortisol. Also involved in carbohydrate and protein regulation. However, most of the cortisone found in the body is formed from cortisol by reversible reaction.

C-reactive protein (CRP): An abnormal protein which appears in the blood during the active phase of many diseases. Raised values occur in bacterial infections, heart and certain cancer conditions. Useful guide to rheumatic disorders and the overall degree of inflammation.

Crohn's disease: Chronic inflammatory disease involving any part of the gastro-intestinal tract from the mouth to the anus. Usually located in the lower bowel. Often causes obstruction and abscesses. Usually treated with steroids.

Cushing's syndrome: Excessive level of cortico-steroids, usually a result of overproduction by the adrenal glands. Overuse of prescribed steroids and over-stimulation by the pituitary gland can also cause the condition. Cortisol is the main corticosteroid hormone and it is usually at a very high level in Cushing's syndrome.

Cytokines: Chemicals produced by immune system cells. Also called inflammatory mediators.

Deep vein thrombosis (DVT): Formation of blood clots in the deep veins, most often in the legs. Treatment is usually a prescription for anticoagulants, such as heparin and warfarin, either by injection (parenteral) or by mouth (oral).

Dehydroepiandrosterone (DHEA): Known also as the 'mother hormone'. Made from cholesterol and released by the adrenal glands, it is the precursor hormone of many steroid and sex hormones.

Deoxyribonucleic acid (DNA): The substance in every cell nucleus that contains the genetic information of each species.

Depression: A persistent state of sadness. Symptoms can include headaches, anxiety and fatigue. Poor immune function and infections are common.

Dessicated thyroid: A source of natural thyroid containing both T3 and T4. Made from pig's thyroid and usually sold as Armour thyroid. It has been in use for well over 100 years.

Diabetes: There are two types of diabetes. Type I is an auto-immune disease, linked to the modern high-carbohydrate diet. People with type I diabetes are insulin dependent. Type II accounts for approximately 90% of diabetics. It is also known as adult or maturity-onset diabetes. High blood insulin in childhood, high-carbohydrate diet and obesity are characteristic pre-cursors of type II.

Dimethylglycine (DMG): An amino acid intermediate. Although not a vitamin, it has been called 'vitamin B-15'. It is a common intermediate of cellular metabolism and is prescribed for CFS, epilepsy, autism, immune support and muscle spasticity. DMG metabolises to the amino acid glycine.

D-ribose: A sugar made from glucose (corn based), a precursor of ATP. With co-enzyme Q-10, D-ribose is prescribed to improve mitochondrial function and CFS.

Dysbiosis: A word used to describe a gradual breakdown of the body's health and balance. 'Dys' means faulty, and 'bios' life or growth.

Dysglycaemia: Disordered blood sugar balance.

Dysmenorrhoea: Painful periods, usually causing both abdominal and spinal pain.

Dyspnoea: Difficult or laboured breathing. Many causes and varieties including heart failure, respiratory (chronic obstructive pulmonary disorder), exertional, anaemic etc.

Dysthymia: Chronic, long-term depression. The symptoms can be mild but may influence the personality of the sufferer. Pessimistic, gloomy, lacking in humour, lethargic and critical are typical characteristics.

Electrolytes: Minerals that are needed to regulate nerve and muscle function; also acid-base balance; found in the body fluids.

Endocrine: Pertaining to internal secretions; applied to organs that release their products into the blood or lymph, such as hormones.

Endocrine axis: Term used to describe the interlinked glands including the pituitary, the thyroid, the adrenals, and the ovaries or testes.

Endogenous: Growing from within or arising as a result of causes within an organism.

Endometriosis: Inflammation of cells from the womb lining that establish themselves outside the womb.

Endorphins: Chemicals in the brain that serve to reduce pain and involve a sense of well-being. They are classed as hormones, being secreted by the anterior lobe of the pituitary gland; they also help support the immune system.

Endoscopy: A medical examination using a flexible tube passed via the mouth (gastroscopy) or anus (colonoscopy).

Enzyme: A substance (protein) that catalyses chemical reactions of various substances without itself being destroyed or altered. Many enzyme reactions occur within cells; digestive enzymes, however, operate outside cells within the digestive tract.

Eosinophils: White blood cells that can ingest bacteria and other foreign cells. They can also attach to and help to kill parasites. Eosinophils participate in allergic reactions and assist destruction of cancer cells.

Erythrocyte sedimentation rate (ESR): The rate at which red cells settle in a tube of unclotted blood. Raised levels are non-specific, but can indicate the presence of inflammation. Of particular value in the diagnosis and monitoring of various rheumatic diseases. The ESR is also used in screening for cancers and infections. C-reactive protein is used for similar purposes.

Essential: In medical terminology this can mean a necessary part of a substance, giving it necessary or peculiar qualities. Also to describe a disease that has no obvious external cause. It can also mean indispensible, required in the diet because the body cannot make it, eg EFAs.

Essential amino acids (EAAs): Amino acids that the body requires but cannot itself manufacture. They must therefore be obtained from food. Nine EAAs have been identified; for children 10 are essential. With famine and protein deficiency, children can develop Kwashiorkor.

Essential fatty acids (EFAs): These are fatty acids that cannot be synthesised by human metabolism and must therefore be obtained via food and drink. There are two EFAs – linoleic acid (omega-6) and alpha-linolenic acid (omega-3).

eu: A term meaning well, good or easily. The opposite of 'dys'.

Euthyroid: Having normal thyroid function.

Exogenous: Developed or originating outside an organism.

Fatty acids: The building blocks of all fats and oils in our body and our food. The chief components of triglycerides, in the blood and the adipose tissue (body fat). Fatty acids are the main components of cell membranes and are involved in construction and maintenance of all healthy cells.

Ferritin: A protein that stores iron in the liver, spleen and bone marrow. Blood ferritin is seen as the best test to assess iron status.

Fibromyalgia (fibromyalgia syndrome or FMS): Defined as 'fatigue with pain'. A common, multi-symptom condition with no definitive test in use to identify the problem. Stress with adrenal fatigue and cellular phosphate excess are currently seen as the chief causes. FMS has also been termed 'muscular rheumatism' or 'fibrositis'.

Fibrositis: See Fibromyalgia.

Folate (folic acid): An important B vitamin (vitamin B-9). It has repeatedly ranked as the number one vitamin deficiency in America. Used to treat CFS, arthritis, post-natal depression and dementia, along with vitamin B-12. Deficiency causes megaloblastic anaemia (pernicious anaemia). It has a controlling influence on blood homocysteine.

Framingham Study: Famous American study started in 1948 and ongoing, set up to investigate the factors that cause heart disorders. Early findings suggested a link with high-fat diets but more recent data has suggested this is not the case.

Free radical: A substance that has lost part of its electrical charge by oxidation. In excess, free radicals can contribute to many illnesses. Free radical sources include air pollution, stress, cigarette smoke, pesticides and burnt foods. Antioxidants reduce the risk of damage from free radicals.

Fructose: Fruit sugar, also found in table sugar, maple syrup and corn syrup, honey and many vegetables. Increasing consumption of fructose as an alternative to glucose is seen as one cause of the obesity epidemic.

GABA (Gamma-amino butyric acid): An amino acid and neurotransmitter usually prescribed to treat anxiety and depression. A nutritional, safe, tranquiliser, non-addictive and without side-effects.

General adaptation syndrome (GAS): A term defined by Hans Selye in his book *The Stress of Life* published in 1956. The GAS consists of three stages: the alarm reaction, the stage of resistance and the stage of exhaustion (eventual death). These stages reflect reactions to exposure to stress.

Geopathic stress: The earth's energy pathways, or fields, can be interfered with or blocked by railway lines, telegraph lines and overhead power lines. The pylons are seen to 'steal' the energy flow. Geopathic stress may be located by dowsing, or by measuring air conductivity and background ionising radiation levels.

Glandular extracts (protomorphogens): Animal glands, prescribed to support the function of equivalent human glands. The glands usually come from the organs of New Zealand cattle and are BSE- and hormone-free. They provide organ specific 'pre-cursor' proteins eg thyroid and adrenal glands, and contain no hormones.

Glucagon: A hormone secreted by the pancreas chiefly to raise the level of blood glucose. It is used to treat diabetic 'hypos'.

Glucose tolerance factor (GTF): A complex molecule that requires numerous vitamins and minerals to support energy production, it comprises chromium, vitamin B-3 (niacin) and other minerals, amino acids and vitamins.

Glucose tolerance test (GTT): A two-, five- or six-hour test, involving frequent blood glucose measurements after the ingestion of 50–100 grams of soluble glucose. The longer tests are of value in diagnosing reactive hypoglycaemia.

Glutathione: An antioxidant used to treat heart disease, asthma and infections; also Crohn's disease and colitis. Provides antioxidant protection to the cellular mitochondria.

Gluten: A protein found in wheat, oats, rye and barley. Gluten intolerance is known as coeliac disease.

Glycaemic index (GI): A measurement giving the glucose and blood insulin levels that are raised by various foods. Glucose is 100 and other carbohydrates are measured in relation to glucose. There is also a GI scale based on white bread. The index has many anomalies and faults and was designed originally to assist the design of diabetic recipes.

Glycogen: The chief carbohydrate stored in animal cells. It is formed from glucose and stored mainly in the liver and muscle-tissue. It can be converted back into glucose to be released into the circulation when needed.

Goiter (or goitre): Enlargement of the thyroid gland causing a swelling in the front of the neck. There are more than 30 types of goiter depending on cause, type, location etc.

Gonads (ovaries): A general term for the sex glands – ovaries in females and testes in males.

Gout: An elevated blood uric acid, often with acute pain, in chiefly the toe joints. Called the 'disease of affluence' and seen as a result of excessive meat and alcohol consumption and obesity. Foods containing purine are usually avoided, purines being the chemical that forms uric acid. The chief culprits are offal-meats, shellfish, pork, duck and beef. The recommended high-carbohydrate diet for gout has been disputed.

Graves disease: Hyperthyroidism with goitre and exophthalmus (protrusion of the eyes).

Growth hormone: A pituitary hormone produced to help the body control how carbohydrates, fats and proteins are used to stimulate growth. Deficiency of growth hormone in children leads to poor growth and short height. In adults, deficiency can cause increased fat, fatigue and poor muscle quality. The hormone is used by some athletes who believe it will increase muscle growth and strength and reduce surplus body fat.

Guaifenesin: An expectorant, prescribed to thin mucous and loosen phlegm. Also known to lower uric acid and prescribed to treat gout. Derived from tree bark, its recent use is to reduce cellular phosphate, calcium and oxalate, thus reducing the symptoms of fibromyalgia.

Gulf War syndrome: A group of symptoms experienced by more than 100,000 American, Canadian and British armed forces personnel in the Gulf War (1992). The cause is controversial and the symptoms include fatigue, insomnia, headache, joint and chest pain, diarrhoea and rashes. Chemical weapons, environmental toxins and the side-effects of vaccines have all been considered as possible causes.

Gut fermentation profile (GFP): This test measures changes in blood alcohol following a glucose challenge. Yeast cells in the gut ferment glucose to alcohol. It involves a single blood test and is principally used to measure candidiasis. The test is provided by Biolab Medical Unit.

Gut permeability test (PEG test): A test provided by Biolab Medical Unit in London to identify a possible 'leaky gut'. The test involves urine measurement and can be done at home.

Haemochromatosis: Accumulation of body iron; usually an inherited disorder in women after menopause. Symptoms can include chronic fatigue and hypothyroidism. Diagnosis is based on the blood levels of ferritin (iron stores) and transferrin (an iron-carrying protein). Treatment is usually bloodletting (phlebotomy).

Haemoglobin (Hb): A pigment found in red blood cells, it is a combination of protein and iron. Its main function is oxygen transport. The Hb is therefore a measure of the blood's oxygen-carrying capacity. It also serves to identify iron-deficient anaemia.

Hashimoto's thyroiditis: The most common cause of thyroiditis. This is inflammation of the thyroid and is thought to be an auto-immune disorder. Many patients with Hashimoto's have other endocrine disorders or auto-immune problems, such as adrenal fatigue, Sjögren's syndrome, lupus and rheumatoid arthritis.

HbAIc (glycolated or glycosylated haemoglobin): A protein in the blood which reflects blood sugar levels over the previous two to three months. It is used to test type I and type II diabetes, and also syndrome X. Normal is currently regarded as less than 20 mmol/mol; poor glucose control as above 20 mmol/mol, and diabetic/syndrome X, above 42 mmol/mol.

Helicobacter pylori: A bacterium that causes gastritis (stomach inflammation) and peptic ulcers. Breath tests can detect it. Treatment consists of a cocktail of antibiotics, ant-acids and protein pump inhibitors.

Herpes simplex: Cold sores are caused by herpes simplex type 1, usually around the mouth, transmitted by kissing and other contact. Recurrent and painful. A genital form is usually sexually transmitted.

Herpes zoster: An acute viral disease thought to be linked to poor immunity and the resurgence of a previous attack of chicken pox. Usually affects the spinal trigeminal nerve. Can be severe in elderly patients.

HFCS (high fructose corn syrup): Also known as maize syrup, glucose syrup, fruit fructose, isoglucose or glucose-fructose. Now accounts for up to 40% of sweeteners in drinks and foods. The use of HFCS is seen as a major factor to explain the current epidemic of diabetes, syndrome X and obesity.

Histamine: A chemical present in all body tissues. Its functions include dilation of small blood vessels, contraction of smooth muscle tissue, acceleration of the heart rate and the increase of stomach secretions. Histamine intolerance (HIT) is a condition caused by lack or reduced activity of an enzyme called diamine oxidase (DAO).

Homocysteine: A metabolite that can increase in the blood and contribute to cardiovascular disease. It can occur from the conversion of the amino acid methionine to the amino acid cysteine. This is usually seen as an inborn error of metabolism. Accumulated blood homocysteine (homocysteinemia) can be reduced by vitamins B-6, B-12 and folate.

Hormone: Powerful chemical messengers produced by the nine major endocrine glands. These, with specialised tissues, produce over 200 different types of hormones.

Hormone replacement therapy (HRT): Replacement of the female hormones oestrogen and/or progesterone. Although chiefly prescribed during or after menopause or hysterectomy, HRT is also prescribed to treat depression, osteoporosis, arthritis, Alzheimer's disease, low sex drive and the pre-menstrual syndrome.

5-Hydroxytryptophan (5-HTP): A precursor of the neurotransmitter serotonin, prescribed to treat anxiety, depression and insomnia. Plant based and side-effect free.

Hyperinsulinism: Inappropriately high levels of blood insulin, also termed 'insulin resistance' or 'syndrome X'. Calories tend to be converted to fat instead of energy. Hypoglycaemia can also result from insulin excess.

Hypertension: High blood pressure.

Hypo-adrenalism: Under-functioning of the adrenal gland, also called adrenal fatigue (see Addison's disease).

Hypochlorhydria: Low stomach acid (hydrochloric acid).

Hypoglycaemia: An inappropriately low level of blood glucose, usually caused by under-functioning of the adrenal glands or insulin excess, as in poor diabetes control or hyperinsulinism.

Hypotention: Low blood pressure.

Hypothalamus: Located within the brain. A vital master control, especially to the pituitary gland, for water regulation and balance, body temperature, biological rhythms and emotions. It has been termed 'the master gland'.

Iatrogenic: A condition resulting from treatment – that is, caused by a health practitioner.

Idiopathic: Defined as arising from within and of unknown cause.

Immunoglobulins (antibodies or Ig): These substances protect the body by attacking bacteria and viruses. They are divided into five classes, known as IgM, IgG, IgA, IgD and IgE. These are defined dependent on their activity and structure.

Insulin resistance: Seen as part of syndrome X and its defining characteristic. High blood insulin is typically a result of inefficiency in the control of insulin, and blood insulin rises in an attempt to balance the blood sugar level. The high-carbohydrate western diet is seen as the main cause.

Intrinsic factor: A glycoprotein secreted by specialised cells in the stomach lining, it is necessary for the absorption of vitamin B-12. Lack of this factor is the cause of pernious anaemia. Porcine-derived intrinsic factor is usually included in vitamin B-12 supplements.

Irritable bowel syndrome: A digestive tract disorder involving a sensitive bowel with alternating diarrhoea and constipation. Other symptoms can include cramping, abdominal pain and fullness, reactions to specific foods, gas, nausea, headaches, fatigue and depression.

Ketosis: The accumulation of keto acids, caused usually by the breakdown of fats in a very low-carbohydrate diet. These keto acids are excreted via the kidneys. Those who follow a low-carbohydrate diet need to drink plenty of water. Any symptoms are usually transient.

Lactase: A digestive enzyme that converts lactose into glucose. Lactase deficiency or lactose intolerance is a common condition in infancy. Treatment involves either the complete avoidance of all milk products, or the use of supplementary lactase taken prior to eating milk products or drinking milk.

Lactic acid (lactate): With oxygen deprivation, the metabolism turns to a back-up energy production system known as lactate fermentation or anaerobic metabolism. This allows lactic acid to accumulate in the tissues causing muscle pain and fatigue. Such a condition can result from prolonged or heavy exercise (eg marathon races). Severe increase in lactic acid (lactic acidosis) can occur in poorly controlled diabetes.

Lactose: Milk sugar made of glucose and galactose.

Leaky gut syndrome: Increased gut permeability, which can allow the leakage of partially digested food into the blood stream. This can lead to specific food intolerances. Chronic gut inflammation caused by *Candida albicans* and other parasites can cause a leaky gut.

Legionnaire's disease: A condition caused by a water-based bacteria and spread via the water or air-conditioning systems in hotels, hospitals, office blocks etc. Symptoms include fatigue, headache, fever and muscle pain. It is linked to pneumonia and can be fatal, but is non-contagious.

Libido: The sex-drive or energy.

Low-frequency sound (LFS or infra sound): Inaudible or infrasonic sound, produced by wind turbines. Symptoms experienced by being close to turbines can include fatigue, insomnia, anxiety, headaches, dizziness, depression, nausea and poor memory and concentration.

Lupus (systemic lupus erythematosus or SLE): An auto-immune condition of the connective tissue, this is a chronic inflammatory disorder that can involve the joints, kidneys, mucous membranes and the walls of the blood vessels. More than 90% of patients are women in their teens to early 30s. The exact cause of SLE is unknown.

Lyme disease: Bacteria that are transmitted to people via infected tick bites, usually deer ticks. Although recognised in Lyme, Connecticut, USA in the 1950s (hence its name), it was also known in Victorian times. It is now the most commonly diagnosed insect-born infection in the USA, occurring in 47 states. Infective ticks are usually present in the summer, in wooded areas. Symptoms include fatigue, aching joints, headaches and fever with chills. Onset is with a large red spot at the site of the bite. This can be 6 inches (15 centimetres) in size. In the UK Lyme disease is principally found in woods and forests where deer can be common. Ticks can also feed on sheep, hedgehogs, foxes and badgers.

Lymphatic system: A huge complex of capillaries, valves, ducts, organs and nodes forming an important component of the immune system. Lymphatic drainage techniques using massage are used to assist drainage of toxins that can accumulate in the lymph system.

Lymphocyte: A white blood cell responsible for specific immunity, including the production of antibodies. The lymphocytes increase to repair cellular damage and reduce inflammation. An increase in the blood count can usually confirm that healing is taking place.

Malabsorption: Poor assimilation of nutrients including minerals and fat-soluble vitamins through the gastro-intestinal tract, or gut. This can occur in many disorders, including leaky gut, diarrhoea, irritable bowel syndrome, gluten sensitivity (coeliac disease), malnutrition, Crohn's disease and candidiasis, and also following surgery.

Melatonin: A hormone, released by the pineal gland, located in the brain that is prescribed chiefly for insomnia and as a remedy for 'jet-lag'. Safety with long-term use has yet to be established.

Menorrhagia: Abnormally heavy or prolonged menstrual periods. This is a major cause of iron-deficient anaemia. (A woman suffering from menorrhagia can lose the equivalent of four to six weeks' dietary iron during one period.)

Metabolic syndrome (syndrome X): A group of symptoms, defined by endocrinologist Gerald M Reaven of the USA as syndrome X or metabolic syndrome, in 1988. The symptoms include high blood insulin, raised blood fats (triglycerides), insulin resistance, raised blood pressure, being overweight and fatigue. Many practitioners blame syndrome X on the western high-carbohydrate diet.

Metformin (bignanide): The first choice drug with overweight type II diabetics. Side-effects include anorexia, nausea, vitamin B-12 deficiency and fatigue.

Mitochondria: Small structures found in all cells. They are the principal sites for energy production and ATP synthesis. Many people see mitochondrial dysfunction as the chief cause of chronic fatigue. Each cell contains approximately 3000 mitochondria.

Monocytes: One of the types of white cell in the blood. They are formed in the bone marrow and transported to areas of inflammation to engulf foreign molecules and cellular debris.

Multiple chemical sensitivity syndromes (MCSS): CFS triggered by a low level of exposure to environmental chemical substances. The common causes include: pesticides, herbicides, food additives, caffeine, alcohol, drugs, cleaning agents and nicotine.

Myalgic encephalomyelitis (ME): Myalgic encephalomyelitis literally means 'inflammation of the brain, with muscle pain' and is a name coined in 1956 for a variant of the CFS family of conditions that was thought to be triggered by a viral infection. Many doctors consider it to be psychological in origin and prescribe anti-depressants and counselling for it. The term ME is being replaced by CFS (chronic fatigue syndrome) in the UK and CFIDS (chronic fatigue immune dysfunction syndrome) in the USA.

Myofascial pain syndrome (MPS): A chronic non-inflammatory condition thought to be related to fibromyalgia, which can affect any of the muscles but chiefly causes pain in the head, neck, and spine. It is often caused by local injuries.

Myxoedema: A severe form of hypothyroidism.

NADH (Nicotinamide adenine dinucleotide): The active co-enzyme form of vitamin B-3 (niacin), also known as co-enzyme 1. It is an essential component of energy production and is a precursor of ATP. It also provides anti-oxidant protection to the mitochondria.

Naturopathy: A system of treatment which recognises that the human body possesses self-curative properties which can resist disease. Naturopathy may include hydrotherapy, nutrition and dietetics, acupuncture, herbalism and homoeopathy. Naturopathic diagnosis is more concerned with establishing why health has broken down than with putting a name to an illness.

Neurotransmitter: Tiny chemical messengers or substances that serve to relay signals across synapses (nerve junctions). Different types of nerves use different transmitters; examples include adrenalin, dopamine, glycine, endorphins and serotonin.

Nitrous oxide (laughing gas): A gas used as an anaesthetic in medicine. Also a recreational drug, which causes a sense of euphoria and a dreamlike state. Side-effects include fatigue and limb numbness.

Non-steroidal anti-inflammatory drugs (NSAIDs): Drugs used to treat rheumatic diseases and inflammatory disorders. They carry a risk of gastro-intestinal side-effects. They are also prescribed for pain. The best known are ibuprofen and aspirin (though the latter is not always classed as an NSAID).

Oestrogen (estrogen): Produced in the female ovaries, this hormone controls the development of the female sex characteristics and the reproductive system. Small amounts are also produced by the adrenal glands. There are up to 20 different female hormones classed as oestrogens.

Omega-3, omega-6 and omega-9: These are the three members of the fatty acid family. The 'omega' number depends on the positioning of double bonds in the molecular structure of fatty acids. Examples of sources are as follows:
- Omega-3 – cold water fish, flaxseed oil, soybean oil and wild game
- Omega-6 – linseed oil, sunflower oil, evening primrose oil, borage oil, blackcurrant seed oil
- Omega-9 – nuts, olives, avocados, sesame seeds.

Ovaries: The two female sex glands.

Oxalate: A chemical that is involved in energy production and is excreted in the urine. Plants such as fruits and vegetables are high in oxalates. Vulvar pain, which is a frequent symptom of fibromyalgia, is thought to be associated with high levels of oxalate excretion. Diets low in oxalates, coupled with the use of guaifenesin, have been found to be of value for treatment.

Oxytocin: A pituitary hormone which causes the muscles of the uterus and milk ducts in the breast to contract to assist milk ejection. It is injected to induce labour in pregnancy and it increases the force of contractions in labour and to control possible haemorrhage after delivery of the placenta. Its role in pregnancy is thought to explain why women with CFS often feel much better when they are pregnant. Non-pregnant women have improved also with oxycitin injections. It increases blood flow to the leg muscles and brain. Its use for CFS remains controversial.

Paraesthesia ('pins and needles'): This generally describes a feeling of numbness, pricking, burning or tingling, usually in the hands, feet or legs, as a result of poor blood flow.

Parathyroid glands: Several small glands (usually four) attached to the thyroid. They secrete the parathyroid hormone which controls bone formation and aids the regulation of calcium and phosphorus.

PCBs (polychlorinated biphenyls): Chemicals used as coolants and electrical insulators, banned by US Congress in 1979 and the Stockholm Convention on Persistent Organic Pollutants in 2001 because of concerns about their causing cancer.

Perimenopause (pre-menopause): Term used to describe the phase before a woman's full menopause. Symptoms can begin as early as age 35 years and continue for up to 15 years. The effects can include depression, fatigue, muscle-joint symptoms, headaches, insomnia, mood swings, osteoporosis, weight gain and loss of libido. Many alternative practitioners view perimenopause as resulting from oestrogen dominance and prescribe natural progesterone. Medical doctors prescribe oestrogen patches or oral contraceptives.

Pernicious anaemia: Anaemia caused by lack of the intrinsic factor that is essential for the efficient absorption of vitamin B-12.

Perrin technique: A physical therapy conceived by Dr Raymond Perrin to treat chronic fatigue. He has defined CFS as a 'structural disorder'. His technique aims to drain toxins from the central nervous system, using specific manual therapy techniques, the main therapy being osteopathy.

Phlebotomy: Puncturing a vein to take blood for testing or to extract blood, as with giving blood or treatment for haemochromatosis.

Phosphate: Inorganic phosphate can build up in the mitochondria of cells, often as a result of kidney malfunction. This is seen by many practitioners as the central cause of fibromyalgia symptoms.

Phyto: Related to a plant or plants.

Phyto-oestrogens: Plant-sourced oestrogens found chiefly in soya, flaxseed, red-clover and black cohosh.

Pituitary gland: A vital 'master gland' in the brain responsible for the control of the other endocrine glands such as the adrenals, thyroid, and testes or ovaries.

Placebo: A 'dummy' medical treatment, prescribed solely for its psychological value. Currently, placebos are part of medical trials, to judge and compare benefits of the trial drug as compared with the placebo.

POPS (persistent organic pollutants): Toxic chemicals also known as 'xenobiotics'. Examples include dioxins, PCBs, aldrin, DDT and dieldrin.

PCOS (polycystic ovary syndrome): A multi-symptom condition including depression, insulin-resistance, infertility, irregular periods, acne, being overweight, and excessive hair growth. The cause or causes of PCOS is controversial. The chief hormonal imbalances involve excessive luteinising hormone and follicle stimulating hormone, which result in high levels of oestrogen and testosterone.

Polymyalgia rheumatic: An auto-immune rheumatic disorder that usually occurs in the elderly. Symptoms include arteritis (inflammation of blood vessels) and severe muscle-joint stiffness that gets worse with rest. Treatment is with steroid hormones.

pH: 'pH' stands for 'potential hydrogen'. It is a scale used to represent the relative acidity or alkalinity of a solution. Neutral is 7.0, below 7.0 is acid and above 7.0 is alkaline. The pH value shows the relative concentration of hydrogen atoms in a solution.

Phosphorylation: A term used to describe recharging in the mitochondria of the cells. The 'battery' (ATP) runs down and becomes ADP. The recharging creates ATP for energy use.

Post-viral fatigue: Fatigue, resulting from and following a viral infection.

Prebiotics: These nutrients are prescribed to provide fuel for beneficial gut bacteria. They assist bacterial balance and improve any disruption of gut permeability. They are termed FOSs (fructo-oligo saccharides) and are to be found in the following foods: onions, asparagus, rye, burdock root, Jerusalem artichoke, banana, sugar maple and chive.

Precursor: Something that precedes something else, such as a substance from which another, more mature or active substance is formed. It can also be a sign or symptom that precedes another sign or symptom.

Prednisolone: A corticosteroid drug that is prescribed to treat inflammation and allergic disorders. It has many side-effects and carries the risk of dependency.

Pregnenolone: An adrenal hormone, known as the 'grandmother hormone'. DHEA, testosterone, oestrogen, cortisol, aldosterone and progesterone are all synthesised from pregnenolone. It is prescribed for depression, rheumatic symptoms, lupus, asthma and adrenal fatigue.

Pre-menstrual syndrome (PMS): A group of symptoms that occur before menstruation. These can include hypoglycaemia with sugar-craving, mood changes, fatigue and an increase in weight resulting from fluid retention.

Probiotics: normal healthy 'friendly' gut bacteria. The big three are acidophilus, bulgaricus and bifidus. These, as supplements, are prescribed in anti-candidiasis programmes and to generally improve gut health and digestive efficiency. They are essential following anti-biotic use.

Proteins: Complex organic compounds containing carbon, hydrogen, oxygen and nitrogen. Proteins are found in plants and animals and consist of 20 different amino acids. They are the main building blocks of the body and the chief component of most cells.

Progesterone: Female hormone that is dominant in the second half of the female cycle. Suppression of hormonal progesterone production is seen as the major cause of oestrogen-dominance symptoms. Natural plant progesterones (phytoprogesterones) are prescribed in the form of hypo-allergenic cream.

Protomorphogens: See 'Glandular extracts'.

Proton pump inhibitors: These are the most potent group of drugs for acid reduction. They are used to treat excess stomach acid and to promote ulcer healing. They can cause many side-effects and are usually regarded as short-term drugs, eg Omeprazole (Losec).

Psychogenic: Produced or cause by psychic or mental factors rather than organic or physical factors.

Psychosomatic: Pertaining to the mind-body relationship; having bodily symptoms of psychic, emotional or mental origin.

Quercetin: A flavonoid anti-oxidant that is a natural anti-histamine, contained in fruit and vegetables. It is prescribed to treat cancers, allergies and heart disease.

Raynaud's disease or phenomenon: Loss of circulation to the fingers, toes or ears and nose with pallor, paraesthesia and pain.

R-binders (cobalophilins): A protein (salivary receptor) that plays a major part in vitamin B-12 metabolism. There are reports of patients with multiple sclerosis symptoms caused by a deficiency of R-binders.

Recommended dietary allowance (RDA): The amount of nutrients, including proteins, carbohydrates, minerals, fats and vitamins recommended as an essential and necessary part of our daily food and drink intake to maintain 'normal' health. These amounts are based on 'average' individual needs and do not always take into account the requirements of the elderly or sick. The optimal blood and tissue levels, nutritional requirements, biochemical individuality, nutrient and drug interactions and other aspects of physiological function, suggest the possibility that many RDAs for vitamins, minerals and amino acids etc are currently too low.

Red cell blood tests: Many blood tests are now red cell estimations (measures of red cell contents rather than of the blood generally). These include mineral profiles, folate, fatty acid profile and essential red cell fatty acids (omega-6/omega-3 ratio). The red cell tests offer more precise information on nutrient status than the traditional tests.

Restless leg syndrome: Constant involuntary leg movement, usually when resting. There are many causes including anaemia, neuritis, magnesium deficiency and varicose veins. Common in the elderly and in pregnancy. Treatment includes folic acid, magnesium, vitamin E and iron.

RSI (Repetitive strain injury): Pain and stiffness, usually in the hands, arms, neck, shoulders or spine, often resulting from regular use of particular muscles and joints. This use may not be initially painful, but over a lengthy period of time can become severely painful. Often occupational and the subject of many work-related injury claims.

Rheumatism: A term used to describe a large group of conditions that involve inflammation, pain and stiffness of joints, muscles and ligaments. These include arthritis, gout, lupus, spondylitis and fibromyalgia.

Ribose: A sugar derived from corn when used as a supplement. ATP is made from D-ribose and D-ribose can also be made from glucose.

Royal Free disease: A term used to describe CFS after an outbreak of sudden fatigue in the Royal Free Hospital in London. Diagnosed in 1956 as caused by mass hysteria.

Seasonal affective disorder (SAD): A mood disorder, triggered by season change and winter light reduction. Many consider that the pineal gland's hormone, melatonin, is the key to SAD treatment and control. This is now disputed as there is evidence that thyroid function can also be reduced in the winter months.

Salicylates: Medicines in use for over 3000 years that are extracted from willow bark, the chief drug being aspirin. They compete with guaifenesin and it is essential to avoid them when using guaifenesin to treat fibromyalgia.

Schmidt's syndrome: A condition with both adrenal and thyroid insufficiency. Symptoms can include fatigue, muscle pain and cramping.

Serotonin (5-hydroxytryptamine): A brain neurotransmitter, also acting as a vaso-constrictor when blood vessels are damaged. Serotonin is a precursor of the hormone melatonin. Prozac and other anti-depressant drugs act by increasing the levels of serotonin.

Short chain fatty acids (SCFAs): These are produced from the fermentation of fibre in carbohydrates in the intestines, examples being acetate, butyrate and succinate.

Sjögren's syndrome: A symptom complex affecting the lachrymal (tears) and salivary glands, causing dry eyes, rheumatoid symptoms and linked to SLE (lupus). The cause is unknown, but it is classed as an auto-immune condition.

SLE: See 'Lupus'.

Sleep apnoea: An absence of spontaneous breathing occurring during one's sleep. The attacks are usually transient and brief.

Somatic: Describing the soma or body; pertaining to the body wall in contrast to the internal organs (viscera).

Statins: A group of drugs prescribed to reduce cholesterol. They are controversial owing to their side-effects. These include fatigue, muscle and joint pain, headaches, constipation and rashes.

Steroid: Anti-inflammatory hormones are in this group and known as corticosteroids. Others in the group include progesterone, DHEA, adrenal hormones, cholesterol and bile salts.

Super oxide dismutase (SOD): An enzyme that offers protection from free radical damage to the brain and the body. It is an anti-oxidant enzyme. It is usually part of liver detoxing formulae. Superoxide dismutase studies form an important component of the Acumen CFS test.

Synacthen test (ACTH): This is seen as the definitive test for adrenal failure (Addison's disease). Cortisol is measured in the blood following an injection of the hormone ACTH.

Syndrome: A set of symptoms which occur together – a symptom complex.

Syndrome X: See 'metabolic syndrome'.

Synergist: A medicine or supplement that aids or co-operates with another or an organ or tissue (eg muscle) that acts in accord with another.

Testosterone: A hormone secreted by the male testes which controls the development of the male sex characteristics and reproductive system. It is important in the maintenance of muscle mass and bone tissue in adult males.

Thrush: Word used to describe oral or vaginal overgrowth of *Candida albicans*, a fungal infection (see Candidiasis).

Thymus gland: An important component of the immune system, situated in the centre of the chest. Its main function is the production of T-lymphocytes. Thymus glandular supplements are prescribed to treat many immune system conditions, including candidiasis, cancer and AIDS.

Thyroid stimulating hormone (TSH): A pituitary hormone, released to stimulate the production of thyroid hormones. Seen by many doctors as the key diagnostic blood test for thyroid status.

Thyroxine (T4): The chief thyroid hormone, which is converted to the active hormone T3 when required. There is 50 times more T4 in the blood than T3.

Total load: A term used to describe how a combination of toxins affects the health, all of which must be taken into account when assessing the causes and treatment of a health problem. Examples apply to environmental factors, domestic and employment stress and nutritional deficiencies. Fatigue is the chief symptom caused by 'total load'.

Toxoplasmosis: An infection caused by toxo-plasma gondi, a single-celled parasite. Diagnosis is usually based on blood tests. Animals can be carriers.

Trans-fats: These have been described as 'toxic fats'. The official term is 'partially hydrogenated vegetable fat' or TFA (trans-fatty-acid). This is a harmful by-product of the hydrogenation process to make solid margarine from liquid vegetable oils. It is currently viewed as potentially a contributing cause of heart disease.

Triglycerides: Triglycerides are the principal fat in human blood. They are bound to protein, forming high and low density lipoproteins (HDL and LDL). Measuring triglycerides in blood can be a valuable test which can provide clues to a possible diagnosis of heart disease, syndrome X, PCOS, strokes, diabetes and obesity.

Triiodothyronine (T3): The thyroid hormone, chemically active at cell level.

Ubiquinone: See 'Co-enzyme Q-10'.

Uric acid: A product of cell nucleic acid breakdown that enters the blood. Uric acid is transformed from purines in food (these foods include anchovies, consommé, herring, asparagus, organ meats, sardines and meat gravies and broths). The blood uric acid also rises when the kidneys fail to eliminate sufficient through the urine. The urate crystals result and are deposited in joints; see 'Gout'. Alcohol also increases uric acid production.

Virus: Minute infectious agents. They can only replicate within living host cells. They are classified according to their origin, mode of transmission, or the symptoms or disorders they produce; they can also be named after the geographical location where first identified.

Vitamins: A vitamin is an organic compound required by the body in limited amounts as a vital nutrient. An organic chemical compound (or related set of compounds) is called a vitamin when it cannot be synthesised in sufficient quantities by an organism, and must be obtained from the diet. General word to describe many substances, they are essential, usually in trace amounts for a healthy metabolism. They may be water or fat-soluble.

Fat-soluble vitamins: Vitamins A, D, E and K.

Water-soluble vitamins: All vitamins except A, D, E and K. Water-soluble vitamins cannot be stored by the body, and need topping up every day.

Vitiligo: A disorder of the skin in which a localised loss of melanocytes leads to smooth white skin patches. The cause is unknown, but it may be an auto-immune condition. Up to 30% of patients also have thyroid disease. Diabetes, Addison's disease and vitamin B-12 deficiency can also increase the risk of vitiligo.

White blood cells (leucocytes): The body's chief defence against infection and inflammation. The percentages of the different cells (differential count) can be used to assist differential diagnosis particularly regarding types of inflammation.

White cell types: Neutrophils, eosinophils, basophils, lymphocytes and monocytes.

Wilson's disease: Hereditary condition in which the liver fails to excrete excess copper. Symptoms include tremors, poor co-ordination and personality changes.

Wilson's syndrome: Named after an American thyroid specialist who considered that many patients with hypothyroidism were unable to convert the hormones T4 to T3, as a result of stress leading to an enzyme deficiency. Many believe that Wilson's syndrome simply comprises the symptoms of depression. Treatment with high dosage T3 is controversial.

Xenobiotics: Any chemical that is normally foreign to a biological system.

Index

Note: bold indicates references in the glossary section.

Note: bold indicates references in the glossary section.

Index

Note: bold indicates references in the glossary section.

Note: bold indicates references in the glossary section.

Index

Note: bold indicates references in the glossary section.

Note: bold indicates references in the glossary section.

Index

Note: bold indicates references in the glossary section.

Note: bold indicates references in the glossary section.

Index

parasites, 64

PCBs, 76

PEG (gut permeability) test, 129–130, 210, **264**

pepsin, 45

   Betain HCl with, 62

perimenopausal women *see* pre-menopausal women

pernicious anaemia, 46–47, 112–113, 118, 186, 187, **272**

Perrin technique, 164–165, **272**

persistent organic pollutants (POPS), 75–76, **273**

pesticides, 76, 77

phlebotomy, 225, 244, **264**, **272**

phosphate (and fibromyalgia syndrome), 58–59, **272**

   removal of excess, 198

phosphorylation of ADP (oxidative), 168, **273**

physical/biological causes (possible evidence), 2, 39–40

   post-viral fatigue syndrome, 219–220

Pickwick syndrome, 93–94

Pilates, 165–166

pituitary gland and hormones, 49, 104, 139, 157, **272**

placebo, 242, **272**

Plenadren, 198

poisons (toxins), chemicals as *see* xenobiotics

pollution

   air *see* air pollution

   persistent organic pollutants, 75–76, 272

polychlorinated biphenyls (PCBs), 76

polycystic ovary syndrome, 67, **273**

polyethylene glycol/PEG (gut permeability) test, 129–130, 210, **264**

polyglandular autoimmune syndrome type II (Schmidt's syndrome), 56–57, **276**

polypharmacy, 235

post-natal depression, 33, 34

post-viral fatigue syndrome, 6, 9, 39, 64, 219–223, **273**

   case history, 221–223

   physical vs psychological cause, 219–220

poverty (low income) and iron deficiency, 43

practitioner selection, 242–243

   see also general practitioners; private doctors/medical practitioners

prebiotics, 129, 164, **273**

prednisolone, 174, 193, **273**

pregnancy, 32–33

   iron-deficiency, 43

pre-menopausal (perimenopausal) women, **272**

   candidiasis, 211

   iron deficiency and anaemia, 41, 42, 44

pre-menstrual syndrome/symptoms (PMS), 30, 33, 34, 54, 65, 66, 104, 134, 221, 239, **274**

   hypothyroidism and, 104

primitive (hunter-gatherer; paleo; Stone Age) diets, 151, 152, 163

private doctors/medical practitioners, 142, 193

private laboratory tests, 107, 110, 117, 142, 185, 244, 245

probiotics, 129, 133, 164, **274**

   candidiasis, 208, 211, 213

   case histories, 19, 211, 213

propranolol hydrochloride, 72

protein, **274**

   digestion, 62

   as oxalate-safe food, 204

   see also high-protein diet

psychological/psychiatric/mental/emotional disorders, 7

   candidiasis symptoms, 59

   in post-viral fatigue syndrome causation, 219–220

   see also specific disorders

psychosomatic rheumatism, 2

puberty, 32

R-binders, 45, **275**

reactive hypoglycaemia, 134, 135, 138

red blood cells (erythrocytes), 48

   low level *see* anaemia

   tests, 275

      mineral, 118

      omega-3 to omega-6 ratio in membrane, 91, 119, 239, 240

      sedimentation rate, 260

      see also haemoglobin

red meat and post-viral fatigue syndrome, 222

relationships, impact on, 4

reproductive system effects of vitamin B-12 deficiency, 48

retirement, old age after, 33

rheumatism, **275**

   in fibromyalgia syndrome definition, 8, 9, 24, 57, 261

   psychosomatic, 2

ribose and D-ribose, **259**, **275**

Royal Free disease, 5, 6, 39, 219, **276**

salicylates, 199–200, **276**

   guaifenesin competition with, 199, 276

   see also aspirin

saliva (hormone tests), 194

   adrenal stress profile, 54, 121, 193–194

      case histories, 16, 19, 178, 186, 212, 216, 225

      female hormonal profile, 120–121

Schmidt's syndrome, 56–57, **276**

serotonin, 19, 56, 175, **266**, **276**

sex (gender), 34

   fibromyalgia and, 34

   symptoms by, 29, 30

   see also females; males

shingles (herpes zoster), 27, **265**

short-chain fatty acids, **276**

   in candidiasis, 213

sick building syndrome, 78

Note: bold indicates references in the glossary section.

Note: bold indicates references in the glossary section.